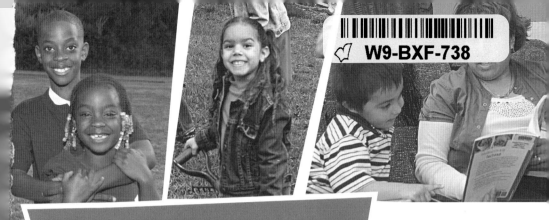

W9-BXF-738

Table of Contents

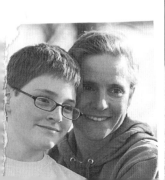

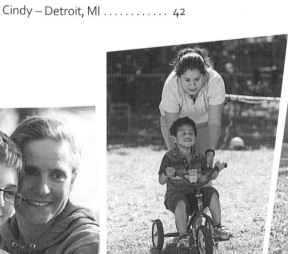

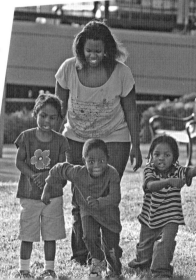

FORWARD

By WILLIAM H. DIETZ, M.D., PH.D.
Director, Division of Nutrition, Physical Activity, and Obesity
Centers for Disease Control and Prevention
Atlanta, GA

Today, roughly one in every three children and teens in the United States is overweight or obese. While there is no single solution to the issue, the Centers for Disease Control and Prevention (CDC) recommends modifying six behaviors to prevent and control obesity.

Behaviors that should be increased include physical activity, fruit and vegetable intake, and breast-feeding. Behaviors that should be decreased include "screen time" (i.e. television viewing, computer time, video games, etc.), the consumption of high energy density foods, and sugar-sweetened beverages.

At the CDC, our job is to focus on policy and environmental changes that support these behaviors. Changing these behaviors within families can also prevent and control obesity.

What is obesity? Obesity is defined as too much body fat. If you have too much fat — especially in your waist area — you're at higher risk for health problems, including high blood pressure, high blood cholesterol, diabetes, heart disease, and stroke.

A person's Body Mass Index (BMI) is calculated from height and weight based on growth chart standards for their age and gender. BMI is used by pediatricians and other medical providers to categorize children as normal weight, overweight, obese, or severely obese. Today, approximately 16 percent of children between the ages of 2 and 19 are obese, and almost an equal percentage are overweight.

FRUITS AND VEGETABLES

Fruits and vegetables contain many vitamins and minerals necessary for health, and more and more studies confirm that fruits and vegetables may also help prevent or control obesity. The sense of "fullness" is regulated by a number of things, including the volume of food consumed. Because fruit and vegetables contain a lot of water, the number of calories they contain is low compared to their volume — they have a low caloric density. The low caloric density of fruits and vegetables also makes them a very good snack for children. In contrast to other foods that need to be limited, children and adolescents can eat as many fruits and vegetables as they choose as long as they are not fried.

PHYSICAL ACTIVITY

Physical activity plays an important role in the control of a number of risk factors for heart disease, and many of these risk factors are associated with obesity. For example, diabetes, high blood pressure, and increased levels of cholesterol are all risk factors for heart disease, and all are related to obesity. Physical activity decreases all of these risk factors.

The Department of Health and Human Services recently released physical activity guidelines for Americans that included recommendations for children and adolescents. The guidelines recommend 60 minutes of daily physical activity, including a mix of moderate and vigorous activity and a mix of aerobic and muscle strengthening activity. Sadly, a recent study indicates that less than 50 percent of children between the ages of 6 and 11 and less than 10 percent of adolescents between the ages of 12 and 19 meet this recommendation.

TV, VIDEO GAMES, AND OTHER SCREENS

Children who watch more television (including for the use of video games) are more likely to be overweight or obese. Furthermore, reductions in television viewing have been shown to reduce weight. Two possibilities help explain why television viewing contributes to obesity. Children who are watching television move less. Their reduced activity may contribute to increased weight gain. Also, there is a clear relationship between the amount of television that children watch, the foods advertised on television, and eating while watching television.

Approximately 25 percent of all 2-year-olds and 65 percent of all children and adolescents have televisions in their rooms. Because children and teens who have televisions in their rooms watch more television, one important way to reduce television time is to keep televisions out of their rooms. In this book, you'll read about a family that did this successfully.

ENERGY DENSITY

As I mentioned earlier, something known as "energy density" has an important effect on fullness. Low energy density foods (foods with a large percentage of water) are filling because of their volume. High energy density foods are foods that are high in fat or sugar, usually have a lower water content, and contain more calories. People who eat a low energy density meal will eat fewer calories. People who eat high energy density foods may consume more calories before they feel full and are more likely to become overweight. Fast foods and desserts are often sources of energy dense foods. Replacing high energy density foods with low energy density foods will make your child feel full faster and reduce the likelihood of extra weight gain.

KEYS TO HEALTHIER LIVING

Increase
Fruits & Vegetables

Increase
Physical Activity

Decrease
Screen Time

Decrease
High Energy
Density Foods

Decrease
Sugar-Sweetened
Beverages

Each chapter contains examples of how moms adopted the behaviors recommended by the CDC to prevent and control childhood obesity. The icons above signify the five behaviors featured in this book. In each chapter, the icons highlighted in the key at the top of each page indicates the behaviors that are discussed in the family's story.

Several of the mothers felt compelled to make changes in their family's diet or physical activity levels in response to their own health concerns or those of their children.

SUGAR-SWEETENED BEVERAGES

Sugar-sweetened drinks include soda and juices that contain 10 percent sugar. Many studies have shown that drinking sugar-sweetened drinks can lead to a greater risk of being overweight and obese. Approximately 15 percent of an average teenager's calories come from these drinks. Calories consumed as sugar-sweetened drinks do not reduce a person's appetite for additional foods. The same is true of juices. The body does not adjust to the sugar in a drink the way it adjusts to a sugar in a solid food. For example, if a person eats sugar in a solid food before a meal, they tend to reduce the amount of calories they eat at that meal. However, if they consume the same amount of sugar in a liquid drink, they do not reduce what they eat to balance the calories in the drink.

BREAST-FEEDING

While none of the stories in this book focus on breast-feeding, it is still an important approach to consider in the effort to prevent childhood obesity. Breast-fed infants have a lower BMI than infants who are fed formula. Any breast-feeding, as well as the duration of breast-feeding, appears to decrease the risk of obesity. How breast-feeding lowers the risk of obesity remains uncertain. One possibility is that when babies are fed formula in bottles, parents often try to get the infant to finish the bottle. In these cases, the baby's fullness may begin to be determined by the parent's concept of what the baby needs to drink rather than the baby's sense of fullness. Over time, these small amounts of overfeeding may lead children to eat or drink more than they would have if they had been allowed to regulate their intake by themselves, and obesity may result. However, mothers who nurse their babies must rely on the baby's cues to determine whether the baby has had enough milk, and therefore may be less likely to overfeed their babies.

SUMMARY

This book presents stories of how families have implemented these strategies to prevent obesity. Several of the mothers felt compelled to make changes in their family's diet or physical activity levels in response to their own health concerns or those of their children. Changes these women made went well beyond their family and prompted changes to increase access to healthy foods and creating safe places to be active in their communities. These are inspiring stories. They demonstrate that children's weight can be controlled, and that these changes can bring families together around healthy living. I sincerely hope that the stories here will inspire other families to make similar changes.

About Dr. Dietz

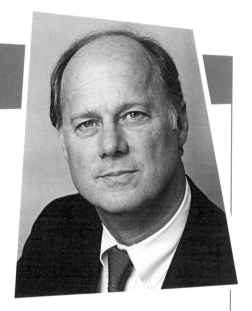

Dr. Dietz is the Director of the Division of Nutrition, Physical Activity, and Obesity in the Center for Chronic Disease Prevention and Health Promotion at the CDC. Prior to his appointment to the CDC, he was a Professor of Pediatrics at Tufts University School of Medicine and Director of Clinical Nutrition at Floating Hospital of New England Medical Center Hospitals. He received his B.A. from Wesleyan University in 1966 and his M.D. from the University of Pennsylvania in 1970.

After the completion of his residency at Upstate Medical Center, he received a Ph.D. in Nutritional Biochemistry from Massachusetts Institute of Technology. He has been a Counselor and past President of the American Society for Clinical Nutrition and was the former President of the North American Association for the Study of Obesity.

In 1995, he received the John Stalker award from the American School Food Service Association for his efforts to improve schools' lunches. Dr. Dietz served on the 1995 Dietary Guidelines Advisory Committee. In 1997, Dr. Dietz received the Brock Medal of Excellence in Pediatrics from the New York Academy of Medicine. In 1998, he was elected to the Institute of Medicine of the National Academy of Sciences. In 2000, he received the William G. Anderson Award from the American Alliance for Health, Physical Education, Recreation, and Dance and was recognized for excellence in his work and advocacy by the Association of State and Territorial Public Health Nutrition Directors.

From 2001 to 2003, he served as a member of the Advisory Board to the Institute of Nutrition, Metabolism, and Diabetes of the Canadian Institutes for Health Research. In 2002, he was made an honorary member of the American Dietetic Association and received the Holroyd-Sherry award for his outstanding contributions to the field of children, adolescents, and the media. In 2005, he received the George Bray Founders Award from the North American Association for the Study of Obesity. In 2006, he received the Nutrition Award from the American Academy of Pediatrics for outstanding research related to the nutrition of infants and children. In 2008, he received the Oded Bar-Or award from the Obesity Society for excellence in pediatric obesity research.

He is the author of more than 200 publications in scientific literature, and the editor of five books, including *Clinical Obesity in Adults and Children* and *A Guide to Your Child's Nutrition*.

Live Well. Eat Well. Be Well.

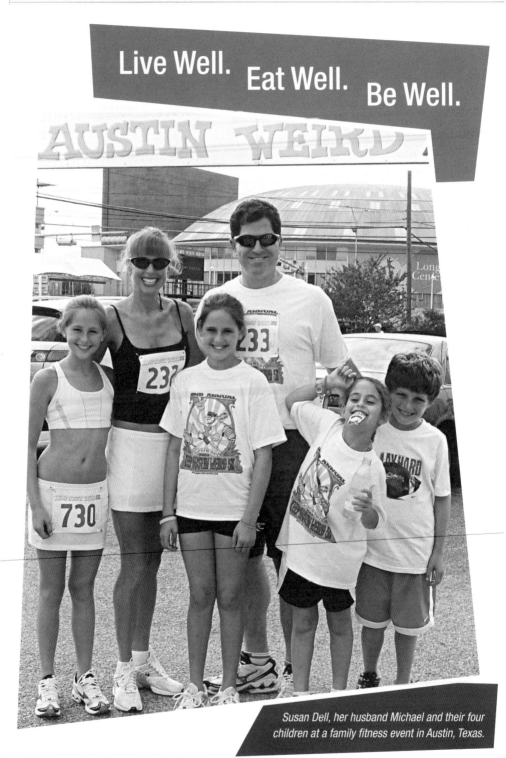

Susan Dell, her husband Michael and their four children at a family fitness event in Austin, Texas.

By SUSAN DELL
Mother
Co-Founder and Chairman of the Board
Michael & Susan Dell Foundation

There are many things a mother wants for her children. She wants them to be happy. She wants them to be educated. She wants them to be kind.

But most of all, she wants them to be well.

In the spirit of that wellness goal, this book was born. As a mother of four, I believe there is nothing more important than giving your children the gift of wellness. The results will last a lifetime.

Nearly 1 in 3 youth, age 2 to 19, are already obese or overweight, and of those, 70 percent will become overweight adults. A child with type 2 diabetes has a decrease of 19 years from their life expectancy. If obesity among kids continues to increase, many believe this current generation of young people will become the first in American history to live shorter lives than their parents. These facts should drive every mother into action.

I have spent the past year finding and interviewing some of the most resourceful mothers in the United States. These are women who believe in doing everything they can to ensure their children embrace a healthy lifestyle. They live in places like New York, Oakland, Philadelphia, Chicago, Detroit, and San Diego. With warmth and enthusiasm, they opened their doors and shared their stories and ideas with the solitary intent of helping other moms.

Many of these women don't have many material possessions, but what they do possess is the creativity and determination to guide their children toward the healthiest lives possible, despite the odds of living in a combat zone of fast foods, sugary treats, and the lure of electronic games and TV. In order to sow the seeds of good health, we asked these inventive women for their tips, plans, recipes, and motivation that help them lead healthy lives.

What I learned is that if it means walking a mile to a farm stand for fresh fruits, they do it. If it means sneaking vegetables into other foods so kids will eat them, they do it. They have even been willing to trigger a community effort to clean up a gang-infested park if it means their kids will have a clean, safe place to exercise.

Many of these moms told us that serious family health issues such as diabetes, cancer, and heart disease were the reasons they decided to make changes in their homes. While these mothers come from all areas of the country, they share the common desire to prevent such health risks in the next generation.

I believe there is nothing more important than giving your children the gift of wellness.

Each mom told me that her No. 1 job in the world was raising happy, healthy children who had options in life. As several of the mothers explained, there are no options if you don't have your health.

All of our moms have faced challenges in their quest to provide healthy foods and opportunities to exercise for their families. In fact, many of them live in tough inner cities where the grocery stores don't even carry fresh fruits or vegetables. Their neighborhood streets are often too dangerous to allow an evening walk for exercise. But that didn't stop them. They found a way.

My heart goes out to the mother who takes two city buses just to buy fresh apples for her daughter. I can't contain a smile when I think about another mom who runs 90 minutes

INTRODUCTION

each night with her two young sons. Bravo!

These moms want to make sure their children have every chance for a good, healthy life. Sometimes they had to make unpopular choices and refuse to give in when their children begged for burgers and fries for dinner. Some had to take the TV remote control out of their kids' hands or even remove television sets from their childrens' bedrooms. Others marched their kids over to the local YMCA to sign them up for exercise classes. Banning soda and salty treats from the home while replacing fattening foods with salads, fruits, and vegetables became a

> *My children wear shirts that say it all: "Go, Mommy, Go!" And the best part of every race is seeing their smiles at the finish line.*

large part of the solution.

Their attempts at good health required some trial and error. For every bowl of carrots that was pushed away with a "yuck," there were those stalks of asparagus that were devoured when served with a healthy veggie dipping sauce. For every child who cried when the cartoons were turned off, there was laughter and cheers when he or she suddenly ran faster from all those nights at the community center and then scored the winning goal during soccer at school.

The changes weren't made overnight, but the changes were made for good.

These moms are incredible to me because their goals don't end at their own front doors. They're great role models to their neighbors and many have made sweeping changes in their communities.

Being a mother means doing whatever it takes to help your children succeed in life. It's about giving your kids the tools to help them form a foundation of good health. My hope is that these children will pass on what they've learned to their friends and, someday, to their own children.

Good health is a priority in my own life and in the lives of my children. My most important roles are those of mother and wife. I'm also an athlete who swims, bikes, and runs in triathlons and marathon races. I've challenged myself to compete in the Kona Ironman World Championships where I swam 2.4 miles in the ocean, biked 112 miles on a hot and windy course, then ran 26.2 miles on pavement, which finally led me to the finish line.

That was the toughest event I have ever done, and what drives me is watching the faces of my incredible family cheer me on. My children wear shirts that say it all: "Go, Mommy, Go!" And the best part of every race is seeing their smiles at the finish line. I've always dedicated my long training sessions and my races to my children and my husband, because they are my inspiration, and I love them more than anything in the world!

Believe me when I tell you that I know how difficult it is to tell a child "no" when they just want pizza or a burger. You're the one who has to find a way to make them choose grilled chicken or a spinach salad instead. And getting 60 minutes of exercise everyday isn't easy either. As a mother, it's all about good health on my watch.

I hope that you share this book with your children and other mothers and that it becomes a springboard for making healthy changes in your family's everyday life.

I wish you all the happiness in the world with your children.

But most of all, I hope that you will all be well.
— *Susan Dell*

About Susan Dell

Susan is co-founder and Chairman of the Board of the Michael & Susan Dell Foundation. The Foundation is dedicated to improving the lives of children living in poverty around the world. With offices in Austin, Texas; New Delhi, India; and Cape Town, South Africa; the Dell family foundation funds programs that foster high-quality public education and childhood health and that improve the economic stability of families living in poverty.

As the driving force behind the Foundation, Susan is dedicated to supporting programs that positively impact children's lives around the world. In the U.S., Susan is specifically focused on encouraging kids to be more physically active and promoting healthy eating, which will help combat the childhood obesity epidemic that is facing our nation. The Foundation has committed more than $500 million to global children's issues and community initiatives to date. The Michael & Susan Dell Foundation focuses its efforts to ensure the programs and initiatives funded by the Foundation are outcome-driven and provide measurable results along the way.

In addition to her charitable work, Susan is the Chairman of the Board of Phi, a New York City-based women's designer collection that made its runway debut in the Fall of 2004. The Phi design philosophy is rooted in the timeless appeal of the confident spirit and state of mind of a modern woman who is both strong and feminine. Phi's creations are available in top designer specialty stores around the world and are often featured in international fashion editorials and seen being worn by celebrities. Phi's flagship store is located in New York City.

Outside of her daily professional responsibilities, Susan competes in marathons, triathlons, and cycling races. Her most recent accomplishments include: fastest woman finisher while setting a new course record for women in the 2007 Kaloko Sprint Cycling Race; fastest woman finisher while setting a new course record for women in the 2006 Sea To Stars Mauna Kea Road Race; setting the record in the 2007 40-44 women's age group for the Cooper Clinic stress test; finished 1st place overall for men and women while setting the course record for women in 2004, a record which she then broke in 2007 in the Kaloko "La La Land" Cycling Race; and she successfully competed in the 2003 Ironman World Championships.

Susan was a member of the President's Council for Physical Fitness and Sports, is a trustee of the Children's Medical Center Foundation of Texas, and a board member of the Cooper Institute in Dallas. She and her husband, Michael, live in Austin, Texas, with their four children.

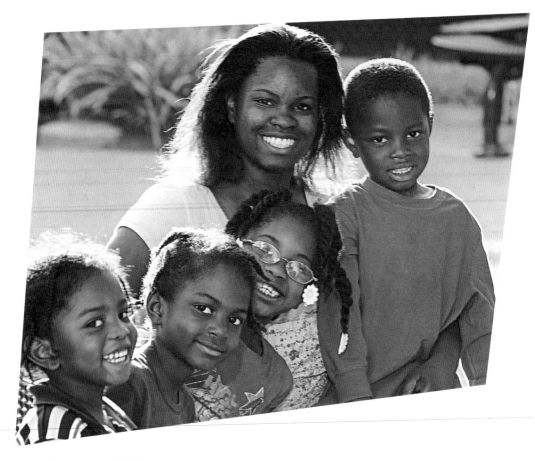

Jamilia – Oakland, CA

A MESSAGE FROM SUSAN

We went to Oakland, California, to find a busy mother of four named Jamilia. Although only 26, she works, attends school, and raises her children, all of them 7-years-old and under. There's Zephariah, 7; Zaniya, 5; Zaire, 4; and Zakari, 3.

What's so great about Jamilia is her major effort to make sure her kids are healthy. It's an issue that's close to her heart. Jamilia burst into tears when we talked about losing her grandmother, Olivia, to diabetes and heart disease. This made Jamilia decide to stop unhealthy habits in her own home.

She also makes sure that her kids get exercise each day in their neighborhood. Jamilia remembers the simple pleasures of running, jumping rope, and riding bikes at top speed, and she has passed them on to her children. It doesn't cost a thing, but the benefits are priceless.

KEYS TO HEALTHIER LIVING

Increase
Fruits & Vegetables

Increase
Physical Activity

Decrease
Screen Time

Decrease
High Energy
Density Foods

Decrease
Sugar-Sweetened
Beverages

"Be ambitious enough to see your child grow old."

That's Jamilia's motto in life. She says it every single day.

Jamilia is a 26-year-old single mother of four, and her kids love to run. Mom races them on the blacktop at school, plays basketball, and rides bikes. She even jumps rope with her daughters. More importantly, she knows that healthy eating and getting exercise are important for a good life.

Jamilia does not want to repeat some of her family members' unhealthy food habits. When her beloved grandmother passed away from diabetes and heart disease, Jamilia made a vow that her children would live healthy lives.

The first step was cutting out all fast foods. Jamilia admits that she would buy burgers and fries for dinner in the old days. As a working mother who also attends school, it was an easy way to provide a quick meal. Now she knows better.

What she wants mothers to understand is that fast foods are unhealthy and can break down strong young bodies, turning them into weak ones. To educate herself, Jamilia looked up the nutritional facts on burgers, fries, and fried chicken on the Internet. She paid close attention to all the calories in these foods. She was shocked to read how full of fat and salt they are.

"You don't want your kids eating grease and salt," she advises. "It's bad for their hearts."

Eating healthy is hard in inner-city Oakland, which suffers from the problems of many cities where the supply of fruits and vegetables is low. In these cities, children are more likely to see guns and violence than a tomato or stalk of celery. Because supermarkets there don't have much of the healthy, fresh foods needed for a good diet, Jamilia made it a family field trip to take a bus to a farmers market so she could buy the freshest fruits and vegetables sold right from the farm, often at lower prices than in the supermarket.

According to the Centers for Disease Control and Prevention (CDC), 1 in 3 individuals born in the year 2000 will develop type 2 diabetes.

After seeing a need in her community, Jamilia is working with community leaders to set up a local produce stand at her school. A first step was organizing a few moms at her school into a group of consumers that would buy these fresh vegetables. She has spoken with local farmers and promised them business, so the farmers are now interested in starting a small stand in Oakland.

Jamilia has had the opportunity to utilize resources such as food stamps to ensure she can provide for her family's basic needs. Jamilia advises that food

Quick Tips

- Involve your kids in planning a weekly menu. Take them shopping and read labels to them.

- Have your kids help you cook. The more involved they are, the more they will want to eat the healthy meals they helped to create.

- Make sure that children do not skip meals. Hungry people can make poor food choices.

- Try at least three or four times to get your child to eat a food. If he doesn't like peas, find a way to put them in other foods he likes.

- Stage a soda-free summer, winter, spring, or fall. Vow to get rid of soda for one season of the year.

stamps should first be used to buy fruits, vegetables, and then lean meats. All junk food should be eliminated.

Jamilia says simple food substitutions can be healthy. For example, she makes fried rice in olive oil using healthy brown rice. She uses ground turkey breast in her spaghetti sauce instead of ground beef. She also adds vegetables, including peppers, onions, carrots, and peas to almost every dish.

When her local grocery store does stock fresh fruits and veggies, she is sure to purchase extras. She cuts them up and freezes them in plastic bags. This way there are always fruits and vegetables on hand. She also makes healthy meals in large portions, freezing some of the meals for quick dinners on busy days.

"Always have something to eat at home," she says. "You won't be tempted to buy fast foods."

Add fruits and vegetables to foods that are cooked or baked. Toss vegetables into pasta sauce, lasagna, casseroles, soups, and omelets.

Breaking bad eating habits formed in childhood is key. When Jamilia was a little girl, her mom put sugar in and on everything. There was sugar added even to the greens and potatoes. Meats like beef and chicken were fried. Now she knows those types of food have to be taken out of the home.

"It's not okay, even if your mama made it that way," she says.

She has a trick for getting children to eat vegetables, even if they don't like

KEYS TO HEALTHIER LIVING

Increase
Fruits & Vegetables

Increase
Physical Activity

Decrease
Screen Time

Decrease
High Energy
Density Foods

Decrease
Sugar-Sweetened
Beverages

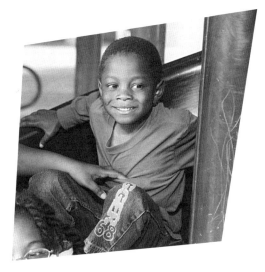

them: She covers them with fruit, even putting a splash of orange juice on top.

Sometimes she will make a homemade pizza with wheat dough. She adds low-fat cheese and tops the pizza with a big smiling face made out of bell peppers for eyes, shredded carrots for the nose, and spinach — what her kids call "the good green stuff" — for the mouth.

Food is only part of a healthy living plan in Jamilia's home. Because she cannot afford a gym membership, Jamilia turned her neighborhood into a gym.

She tells her kids to jump rope or do cartwheels. She'll have them compete to see who can jump the highest or do the most jumping jacks. Sometimes it's as simple as running in an open field. At area schools, she plays basketball or has her kids ride bikes in the school playground.

Jamilia even finds small grassy areas to play tag. She loves to play pretend games that include exercise. She will tell her children to pretend that they're at a big baseball park playing in the major leagues and has everyone run the pretend bases.

Then she offers prizes. The winner gets to choose his favorite activity or pick her favorite healthy breakfast the next morning.

"Change doesn't happen overnight," says the Oakland mom. "But the smallest changes you make with your health habits can make a big difference.

"I want to be there to see my children grow old. I want to see their children," she says, smiling. "I want us to live a long, happy life."

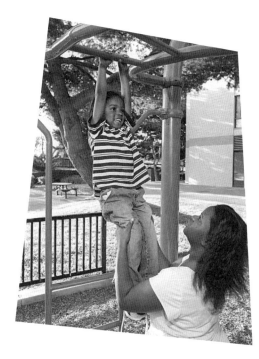

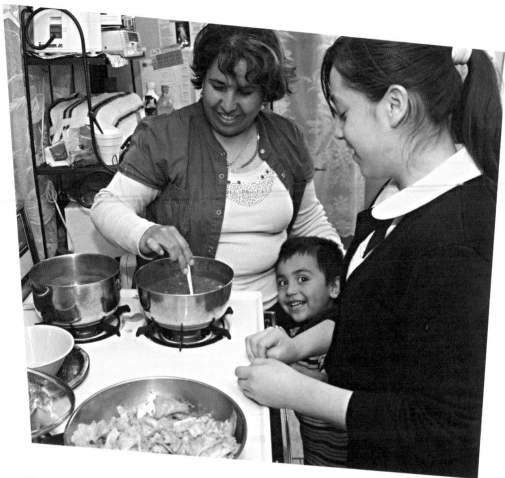

Rosa – Chicago, IL

*T*here are mothers who lead with words and others who believe that actions speak even louder. Rosa is an inspiring mother from Chicago who is showing her children the way to good health.

Rosa told me that more than anything in the world, she loves her husband, Romero, and children Evon, 12; Evelyn, 11; Romero, 9; and Juan, 3. But a severe bout of depression almost knocked out this mom. Soon, her weight reached more than 200 pounds. Rosa was forced to rescue herself through a neighborhood nutrition class that changed her life and the health of her family.

She lost enough weight to drop from a size 22 to a size 8 and now has boundless energy. Her children saw their mother shrinking and were excited about the changes they saw in her. Rosa went from being a mom who used to just sit all day long to one who can't sit still.

Increase
Fruits & Vegetables

Increase
Physical Activity

Decrease
Screen Time

Decrease
High Energy
Density Foods

Decrease
Sugar-Sweetened
Beverages

It was a bit of a battle when a Chicago mom named Rosa decided to change her family's eating habits, especially when her four children decided to stage a revolt.

When Mom served fruits and vegetables instead of pizza and fries, she heard the battle cries.

In part because they lack access to healthy food and sports facilities, children from lower incomes are more likely to be overweight or obese.

"My kids would yell, 'We don't like it. We don't like it!'" Rosa remembers.

But in every battle, there is a general on the front lines, and, in this case, mom was clearly in charge.

"I said, 'I'm doing this for your health. I'm doing this because it's good for you,'" Rosa explains.

Words weren't enough in her stubborn family's case, and Rosa knew her situation required some outside help. She was suffering from high blood pressure and very high cholesterol levels. She also had a serious case of postpartum depression following the birth of her youngest child, and her eating was out of control. She knew that in order to see her children grow up, she needed to make some real changes.

A funny thing happened when this mom dropped 60 pounds. Her children were amazed and wanted to become healthy, too.

Changing their lifestyle involved parting ways with a beloved family member — the living room sofa. Rosa didn't throw it out.

She just stopped spending so much time on it watching TV.

There was a time when Rosa was so out of shape and tired that she never wanted to get up from the couch, and her kids often joined her for hours of just doing nothing. Rosa's pediatrician warned that her 12-year-old son was also suffering from high blood pressure. The boy was also having breathing problems.

"I would fall asleep and just let life pass me by," says Rosa, for whom the simple acts of standing or walking were an effort that left her breathless. She knew that she needed some outside help to save her family — and pronto.

Three years ago, she forced herself to leave the couch and attend a local Chicago nutrition class. That single act literally changed the course of her life. Now, Rosa tells other moms to check newspapers and the Internet for local nutrition courses and seminars. There are many free resources that offer useful tips, support systems, and inspiration. Rosa's nutrition teacher helped put together a healthy eating plan for her and her kids. The idea that she had a real plan made Rosa's spirits soar.

"I came home and danced with my children for the first time in a long time. I had hope," Rosa recalls. "I heard the kids yell, 'Mom is up! She's happy! She's even singing!'"

Rosa's new eating plan for her family

- Limit screen time to one hour per day.

- Eat three small meals and two snacks a day.

- Know that kids "sneak eat." Get rid of all temptations in the house.

- Offer fruit as a sweet snack — your children will grow to love it.

- Explain calories and saturated fats to your children. Make a game of avoiding too many calories and limiting bad fats at each meal.

- Reduce salt at the table and during cooking for good health.

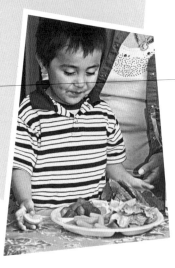

includes eating five times a day in the form of three full meals and two snacks. The snacks consist only of fruits or vegetables.

Early on, even Rosa resisted eating some healthy foods and thought her children felt the same way. But she knew no one in her home would ever eat the new foods on her food plan if she didn't try them first. She knew she had to lead by example.

Rosa soon realized that she couldn't continue to have unhealthy foods in her home. If they were available, her son would choose those items instead of following her meal plan.

Children who are overweight are more likely to suffer from all kinds of health problems — including type 2 diabetes, sleep disorders, and high blood pressure.

As time went on, she taught all of the older children to read labels. She was used to just grabbing products off the grocery store shelf because they looked appetizing. These days she tries to avoid saturated fats and too much salt.

She follows the government-suggested Food Guide Pyramid for portion control and recommended servings per day of lean meats, fruits, vegetables, and grains. Everyone drinks plenty of water each day, and avoids sugary juices.

The new food plan can be a little costly, but Rosa sees the expense as a necessity.

"I say everything in life has a cost, but your health is something you can never put a price tag on," she stresses. "A dollar difference is not worth your life."

She is now happy to report that her oldest son's blood pressure is normal. All of her

KEYS TO HEALTHIER LIVING

Increase
Fruits & Vegetables

Increase
Physical Activity

Decrease
Screen Time

Decrease
High Energy
Density Foods

Decrease
Sugar-Sweetened
Beverages

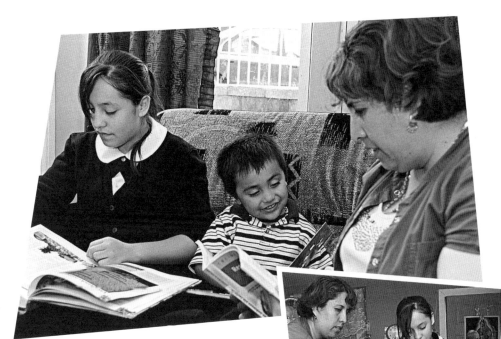

children recently received perfect checkups from the doctor.

She spreads the word on health in her Chicago neighborhood, and other mothers ask Rosa to come into their homes to help them make similar lifestyle changes. Her daughter recently gave a presentation in school about healthy eating, bragging that her mother now has enough energy to dance and play on the floor with her children. Rosa even chases them through the deep Chicago snow banks during the winter.

For her own health, she walks at least 60 minutes a day. Quite often her children will be striding by her side. At home, they turn on music and dance around their apartment.

Sometimes they even drag out her old size 22 pants, a big difference from the size 8 she now wears. The pants are a reminder of how far Rosa's family has come on their journey toward good health.

"Life is our greatest treasure," Rosa says. "I also know that my children are proud of me, and that's the best feeling in the world."

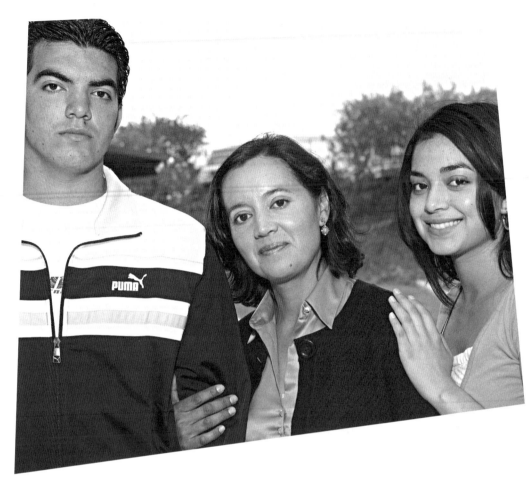

Xinia – San Diego, CA

I love a mother who takes charge and that's what San Diego's Xinia did when she personally asked local restaurant owners and chefs to put healthier foods on their menus. The El Salvador native is a role model to her teenage daughter Xinia, 19; and son Felix, 17. She is also trying to make life better for her entire community. She even helped raise money to completely overhaul a depressed local park. This mom doesn't take no for an answer!

Xinia also believes in real foods. She grew up eating fresh vegetables from local stands. The foods would go from the ground to her plate. Xinia was taught this is the healthiest way to eat and tries to make sure that what she feeds her own children doesn't come out of boxes.

This mom has my respect because she makes sure her kids combine the healthiest diet with daily exercise.

KEYS TO HEALTHIER LIVING

Increase
Fruits & Vegetables

Increase
Physical Activity

Decrease
Screen Time

Decrease
High Energy
Density Foods

Decrease
Sugar-Sweetened
Beverages

Xinia is a mother who knows that one person can change everything.

Unhappy when she saw how many unhealthy menu items were offered at popular local restaurants near her San Diego home, she called and visited the eateries to ask owners and chefs to serve healthier foods instead of ones of the fried variety. So many slammed the door in her face that the mother of a teenage daughter and son was surprised when some of them actually listened.

Now some of those restaurants are serving fruit cups, whole-wheat sandwiches, lean turkey and chicken, and low-fat options. Many added a whole list of healthy options.

"Mothers need to ask for what they need for their children," Xinia says. "It doesn't hurt to have your voice heard. It can help everyone if you speak up."

This driven mom lives in a home full of sunshine where she always has a big bowl of mixed fruits on her kitchen table.

Xinia says that healthy living begins in your kitchen. For starters, she believes that what goes on your child's plate at every meal should look like a rainbow.

The general rule is that colorful, natural foods are usually free from artificial ingredients and packed with many vitamins and nutrients. Eating them regularly may even prevent obesity and other diseases like the common cold and the flu by building up your immune system.

Think about a ripe red apple, a deep green pepper, or a bright orange. Blue and purple foods like blueberries and eggplant and deep yellow or red foods are also antioxidants. Orange foods are packed with vitamin C, which helps kids resist colds and infections. Dark green leafy vegetables like kale, spinach, and collard greens contain omega-3 fatty acids. These help build healthy cells in your body.

"The rule is simple: Each time you add a color, you add health to your meal," Xinia says.

At home, Xinia tries to be creative when making different dishes. Long ago, her kids

If you eat out, try to avoid fried food and order items such as lean meats that are grilled or baked, steamed vegetables, and whole grains.

didn't like steamed vegetables, so Xinia put a little bit of low-fat cheese on the top of them. It makes them more appealing to kids. Scrambled eggs are even tastier with some sautéed veggies in them.

Xinia even found substitutions for her favorite Latin recipes. She makes vegetarian quesadillas with whole-wheat tortillas, onions, red peppers, corn, cilantro, and a whole medley of veggies. She tops them with low fat cheese.

Rice is popular in Latin dishes. But it is a starch with little nutritional value. So Xinia makes sure to add tomatoes, zucchini, peppers, mushrooms, or onions to her rice in order to add vitamins, fiber, and minerals.

Quick Tips

- Eat foods that are colorful — the more the better. These have the most vitamins and nutrients.

- Eat foods that are ripe and in season. The food will go from the ground to your kitchen table.

- Don't buy unhealthy snacks like potato chips and candy bars. If your children don't find it in the house then they won't be able to eat it.

- Remember this rule: Everyone needs to exercise every day.

- Exercise could include walks, dancing, and even dropping down on the living room floor during commercials and doing sit-ups and push-ups. Turn on a CD and dance around the living room.

- Buying fresh fruits and vegetables costs much less than doctor bills!

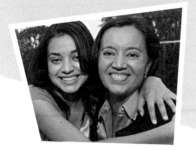

She even chops fresh garlic and slices her own fresh vegetables to put into dishes. "Sometimes, I will go to three supermarkets to make sure my children are eating the freshest fruits and vegetables," she explains.

Over a 15-year study, adults who ate fast food more than twice a week gained 10 pounds more than those who ate fast food less than once a week.

Even when some of the foods are expensive, they are cheaper than doctors' bills. So she's willing to make the sacrifice.

The key for this mom is that her children eat fresh foods. Foods in a can or box often contain chemical additives. For example, fruit in cans often contains high fructose corn syrup (sugar) and include chemicals to preserve the fruit. Some canned vegetables contain extra salt (sodium) for flavor and are therefore a less nutritious choice.

Xinia loves to make steamed chicken with veggies on the side. She covers both with a homemade tomato sauce. And Xinia says any mom can make homemade sauce. You just need to boil a few tomatoes, mash them up, and add some garlic, onions, and spices. She also cuts out some of the fat by buying lean meats.

When it comes to snacks, Xinia is the boss. She absolutely refuses to buy chips, candy, or cookies. Of course, her kids have complained, but mom stays firm. She just ignores their protests and offers fruits and nuts as snacks. Her children eventually eat the healthier foods because there are no other choices.

She cautions moms to really know what's healthy and not. For example, she checks

KEYS TO HEALTHIER LIVING

Increase
Fruits & Vegetables

Increase
Physical Activity

Decrease
Screen Time

Decrease
High Energy
Density Foods

Decrease
Sugar-Sweetened
Beverages

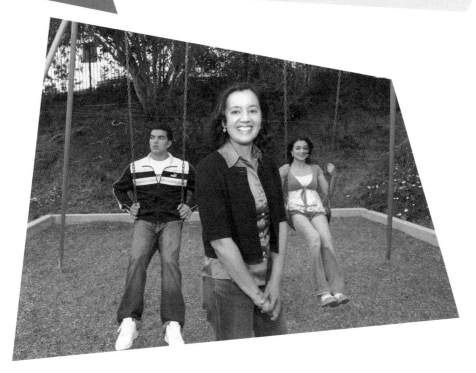

her juice labels. Even when it says apple juice, it's not always 100 percent juice. It might only be 10 percent juice.

Beyond making sure her children are eating the best foods possible, Xinia tells her children that they must find time every single day for physical activity. It's like brushing their teeth or eating. It's a necessity of their daily schedule. She walks with her husband for an hour each night. Her daughter Xinia takes dance classes, including hula lessons. Her son lifts weights at home and does push-ups on the living room floor.

"We encourage 60 minutes of regular exercise a day for children," Xinia says.

Xinia also works with the University of San Diego State Foundation and the Network for a Healthier California by holding community seminars on nutrition, exercise, and healthy living. It's a great way for her to pass on her know-how to other moms.

A woman who practices what she preaches, she also helped revamp a neighborhood park with the help of other moms. They raised an amazing $400,000 for the project by asking for state funding. A once-dilapidated piece of land, the park now has new playground equipment and trimmed grassy areas for children to play baseball and soccer.

"As a mother, it's your job to make sure your children have every chance in life. That begins with health," she says. "I can't think of a better gift to give your children than strong bodies and minds."

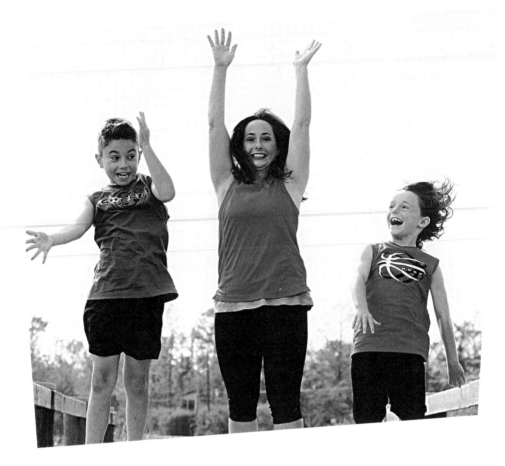

Ashley – Houston, TX

A MESSAGE FROM SUSAN

We traveled just outside the city of Houston to find a special mom named Ashley. Ashley is the mother of two adorable little boys, Avery, 9; and Julian, 7. As with many families, the idea to get healthy began with little steps. First, Ashley decided to run in a local 10K race and enlisted the help of her father who put together a training program they could do together. Sadly, her dad had to drop out due to an injury, but Ashley pushed on and ran her race. Her sons were in the stands and couldn't wait for Ashley to cross the finish line. Why? They wanted her to start training them! Ashley started them with a few laps around the block every night after dinner. This family put one foot in front of the other until they were running together for more than an hour and a half each night. The simple act of running produced results so stunning that the entire family was impacted in breathtaking ways — as I'm sure you will be after reading their story.

KEYS TO HEALTHIER LIVING

 Increase Fruits & Vegetables

 Increase Physical Activity

 Decrease Screen Time

 Decrease High Energy Density Foods

 Decrease Sugar-Sweetened Beverages

There was a major fan reaction when a Houston mother named Ashley ran her first 10K race.

There were more than 1,000 people in the stands. But the ones yelling the loudest were her young sons Avery, 9, and Julian, 7, who screamed, "Win, Mom! Win!"

Ashley didn't cross the finish line first, but what happened thanks to running was better than getting a first place ribbon.

In the marathon called life, her entire family is winning.

Ashley insists that she wasn't born to run. Neither were her children.

"Never in my wildest dreams did I think that running could change everything for my family — but it did," she says. "The impact has been amazing."

She began running thanks to her own father's suggestion and his training. Her Dad was going to run in that 10K with her, but dropped out when he injured his foot. Ashley followed in his footsteps and became a loving and wise trainer for her own kids.

Soon her sons were pounding the pavement with her every night. The results were wide-reaching, to the point that her oldest, who had always struggled with hyperactivity and behavior issues, suddenly was a calmer child.

"I knew that Avery was different," says his proud mom. "When we went to kindergarten, he was in so much trouble every day. I didn't know what to do."

Ashley blamed herself when teachers told her it was probably ADHD. She knew the next step would be for experts to suggest medicating the boy.

Ashley just shakes her head because she was not in favor of using medication as a solution. "All I knew is that I had a very active little boy who didn't like to be at a desk for several hours a day," she says.

According to the Physical Activity Guidelines for Americans issued by the U.S Department of Health and Human Services, children should aim for at least 60 minutes of moderate physical activity every day.

The family tried different behavior modification techniques, but nothing changed Avery's ultra-energetic behavior.

Running is the one thing that worked with this young boy. "This is the first time that I've felt like there is nothing wrong with my child," Ashley says. "This feeling started when we began running."

Avery smiles when asked about how his life is different now.

"A long time ago, I had bad grades. My behavior wasn't so good," Avery says. "Now, for some reason, running has switched my brain. I get good grades now, and I never get in trouble anymore."

For almost no money, Ashley insists that any family can begin a running program. This family started by putting on some

Quick Tips

- Find a beautiful spot to run outdoors, if possible.

- Devote 20 minutes and jog slowly to begin. Add two minutes to that time each week.

- Don't run on a full stomach. Allow at least an hour after dinner for your food to digest.

- Set realistic goals where you progress slowly.

- Run at a speed where you can still talk or even tell stories.

- Teach your children how to set physical goals, then help them stay motivated to reach those goals.

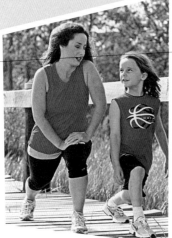

jogging shoes and running for 20 minutes around their neighborhood. The boys did a couple of laps around the block, running as quickly or as slowly as they felt comfortable. There was no pressure. They could stop and start. They just couldn't quit.

"I motivated them by holding them back.

Regular physical activity can help you maintain your weight, keep off weight that you lose, and help you reach physical and cardiovascular fitness.

You don't want them sprinting and winded," Ashley says. "You don't want them to get too tired. I wanted them to go at a steady pace."

Soon, the boys were easily running three to five miles. It was even a bit of competition with the boys trying to out do one another. Mom noticed that there was also teamwork between her sons.

"If one wants to slow down, the other says, 'Come on! You can do it! Follow me!'" she says. "They cheer for each other."

Ashley says that the nightly exercise ritual takes a little bit of planning. This busy teacher makes sure her family eats dinner by 5:30 p.m. They wait a bit for their food to digest and then hit the pavement. She advises not to run just after you eat. This family waits for at least an hour.

Her family runs about five nights a week for an hour and a half now. They eat healthy salads and lean meats, but have some treats. The rule is not to eat too much because it will affect your running.

The time outdoors together has also meant some wonderful family bonding. Avery went from having Us — or unsatisfactory grades — on his report

KEYS TO HEALTHIER LIVING

Increase
Fruits & Vegetables

Increase
Physical Activity

Decrease
Screen Time

Decrease
High Energy
Density Foods

Decrease
Sugar-Sweetened
Beverages

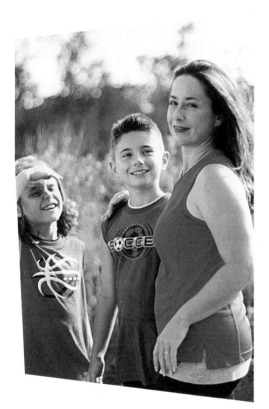

about college. "Have you ever heard a seven- and a nine-year-old sit around talking about getting track scholarships to college?" she asks with a smile. "Running has taught my kids about having a goal — and striving to achieve that goal."

Mom couldn't be more pleased with her sons.

"I love these boys deeply. They're my life. There is nothing more that I want in this world than for them to be the best that they can be and have the happiest life they can have. It's my job to give them those tools now," she says. "Running has been one of those tools."

Avery says that Mom is the best trainer. "When I feel like quitting, she keeps me motivated," he says. "Mom tells me never to stop."

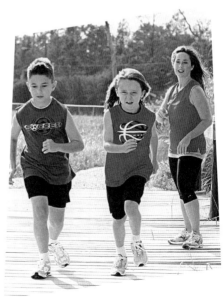

card in all 11 categories, to having 11 Es, which are excellent marks.

"We didn't do anything different at home except run three to five miles a night," Mom says.

Julian holds a gold medal in his hand from a local fun run. "I was the first one to pass the finish line! I even beat the third graders!" he says with pride. "I'm going to run forever!"

The family's routine has also allowed the boys to do better at other athletic endeavors like soccer. Her sons even talk

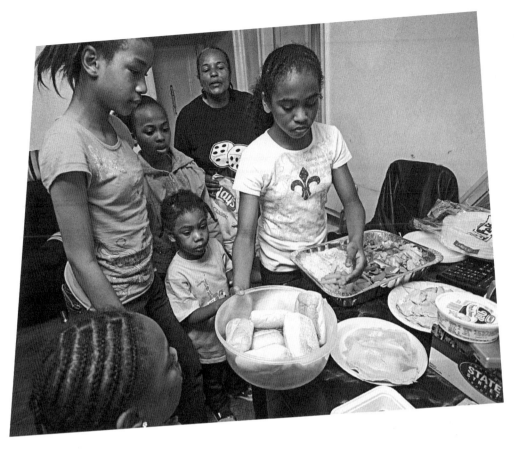

Debra – New York, NY

A MESSAGE FROM SUSAN

It's tough to figure out which is bigger — Debra's heart or her dining room table. A resident of New York's Harlem, Debra is a social worker and single mom to daughter Giovanni. Just two years ago, Giovanni reached her 10th birthday, but looked like a six-year-old. Doctors told this mom that her daughter had stopped growing, and it was heartbreaking for her. The reason was a lack of vitamins and minerals in her body. The solution to the problem would be found on a plate served with love.

Debra began to notice that other children in her building also looked unhealthy. Their mothers worked two or three jobs and weren't home much to cook meals. Debra took it upon herself to open her home and her kitchen. Each night, she serves dinner to upwards of seven children who lovingly call her "Auntie." Debra has ingenious ways to help children get what they need to grow strong and be healthy.

KEYS TO HEALTHIER LIVING

Increase
Fruits & Vegetables

Increase
Physical Activity

Decrease
Screen Time

Decrease
High Energy
Density Foods

Decrease
Sugar-Sweetened
Beverages

Debra is a mom on a nutrition mission each night. She is not a trained chef, but the Harlem native is a savvy parent. Debra believes in healthy, home-cooked meals that can really be stretched.

She is on a limited budget, yet sets her table for 12. It doesn't have to be this way because Debra is a single mom with just one daughter. But this social worker can't stand to see children suffer, which is why 10 kids from her building have been eating dinner at Debra's for more than a year.

Debra feels she has no choice but to open her heart — and table — to kids needing a boost in nutrition.

She noticed kids in her building who had no energy. Some were small for their ages because their bodies weren't growing and others were overweight. Debra went to their mothers and simply asked if these kids could come over for dinner … every night.

"I couldn't allow these children to eat poorly anymore. These kids were eating a steady diet of fried chicken wings from a takeout place, pork-fried rice, French fries, and soda. One mother fed her children that exact meal for breakfast, lunch, and dinner for two whole years," Debra explains.

In Harlem, it's very difficult to eat healthy. A lot of parents work as many hours as possible to survive. You can't buy fruits and vegetables easily because the corner markets don't carry them. There are children in this area who have never eaten a salad.

Debra is a wonder because she will go to any length to act as a healthy-food fairy godmother.

She takes buses to faraway stores and farmers markets to buy fresh fruits and vegetables. She makes meals from scratch. Her mantra is to serve her daughter and the other children the freshest, healthiest foods possible so they can grow to be strong individuals. She even coaches other moms in her building and gives them healthy cooking tips.

> *When reading food labels, pay close attention to the amount of calories, fat, sugar, and sodium in each serving.*

Debra's bag of magic also includes clever ways to get the kids to eat what's right for them. Her approach is to make eating fun for children.

First, she appeals to tiny taste buds. Knowing that children love anything sweet, she puts a little bit of honey or natural maple syrup over vegetables. Debra got rid of boxed breakfast pastries that kids love. Instead, she now serves homemade wheat pancakes full of bits of natural chocolate. She has a special "appetizer," a dip made with yogurt and honey, which she surrounds with fresh vegetables — perfect for dipping.

Debra knows how to deal with stubborn dinner guests. When the kids didn't want to eat skinless turkey dogs because they weren't "real hot dogs," Debra got creative. She got out her sewing needle, sterilized

Quick Tips

- Try to buy as many fresh fruits and vegetables as possible — avoid processed fruits and vegetables that contain added sugar, salt, or sauce.

- Frozen vegetables are good alternatives in winter months.

- Make special dips with a little honey or natural maple syrup. Kids enjoy dipping their veggies!

- Think of fun games to do with food like veggie necklaces or making a forest out of your veggies and eating all the trees.

- Put salad fixings in little bowls — carrots, celery, lettuce, peppers, tomatoes, etc. Ask each child to use at least four things in their salad. Stick with low-fat dressings or homemade ones.

- Avoid foods filled with fat and sodium by reading food labels.

it, and then grabbed some thread to make "necklaces" out of cooked turkey dogs and raw vegetables. She's made similar "necklaces" out of everything from shrimp to fresh fruit.

One of Debra's "regular customers" wouldn't eat his broccoli so Debra appealed to his love of fairy tales to get him to try it. She stood little pieces of broccoli up on a plate, creating "trees" in a magical forest. The boy — pretending to be a brave prince — had to eat the "trees" in order to save the princess. In five minutes, the broccoli was gone.

Debra's fight to save children comes from a personal place. Her own daughter was starving, and this kind and caring mom didn't even know it. Giovanni ate plenty of food each day. But what she ate was

According to the American Heart Association, the estimated calories needed by children range from 900 per day for a 1-year-old to 1,800 per day for a girl between the ages of 14 and 18 and 2,200 for a boy between the ages of 14 and 18.

severely lacking in vitamins and minerals. "I gave my daughter what she wanted to eat — not what she needed," Debra says.

Giovanni's body stopped growing at age six. She was a frail girl who had thin bones. Exhausted or sick all of the time, she would catch every flu bug or cold around. She even had pneumonia three times one year and broke her arm several times because her

KEYS TO HEALTHIER LIVING

Increase
Fruits & Vegetables

Increase
Physical Activity

Decrease
Screen Time

Decrease
High Energy
Density Foods

Decrease
Sugar-Sweetened
Beverages

bones were weak.

After administering various tests, doctors told Debra that her daughter was severely lacking in nutrition. She was deficient in important vitamins, which were not entering her system. Her daily diet included fast foods and greasy meals from a local Chinese takeout restaurant. Her doctor gave Debra a list of healthy food options — lean meats, skinless chicken, fish, fruits, and vegetables — that Giovanni needed for healthy growth. She was also told to buy as much fresh produce as possible.

Giovanni's new meal plan would include whole-wheat pancakes, eggs, or waffles for breakfast. For lunch, Debra was told to make Giovanni healthy sandwiches with fresh meats and low-fat cheeses along with fruits and vegetables. Dinners would also become a new adventure of fresh vegetables, salads, grilled lean meats, and skinless chicken plus a few surprises. She wasn't allowed to eat white bread, fried foods, or drink sugary sodas.

A strange thing happened. After exactly one month of healthy eating, Debra remembers that Giovanni walked into the living room carrying her three new pairs of summer shoes, which had been bought a month earlier. They were much too small! All of sudden, she was growing … and growing.

Now Giovanni runs, dances, and doesn't slow down for a second. Her grades have improved. She sprints out of bed in the morning and races to the dinner table each night. She rarely gets sick. Each night, she eats healthy dinners with her friends who call Debra "Auntie."

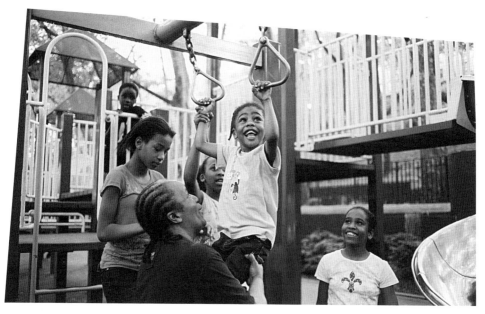

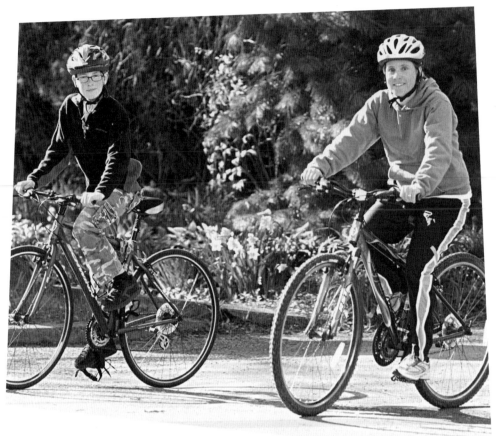

Angie – Harrisburg, PA

Angie is a mother living in Harrisburg, Pennsylvania, who has found a way to make her 12-year-old son, Tim, incorporate exercise and good eating habits into his everyday routine. A runner who is about to adopt three more children with her second husband David, she also had to teach her son what not to eat when he's visiting his dad on weekends. This is a major challenge for so many families. In this case, Tim's dad likes to eat out and go to fast food restaurants. Mom found amazing ways to cope with the fact that what her son is eating isn't always in line with her healthy plan.

Through his mother's urging, Tim has also discovered ways to get daily exercise without joining a school team. Best of all, Angie has found tips that all parents can use to ensure their kids keep a healthy eating mindset no matter what's on their plates.

KEYS TO HEALTHIER LIVING

Increase
Fruits & Vegetables

Increase
Physical Activity

Decrease
Screen Time

Decrease
High Energy
Density Foods

Decrease
Sugar-Sweetened
Beverages

Angie's son, Tim, is a typical 12-year-old who loves cartoons, the Internet, and hanging out with his dog, Haley. But he's not competitive and has no interest in joining a school sports team.

"To be honest, I like to run around. I just don't want to compete with other kids," Tim says. "So, I don't play sports. I just want to play with my friends."

academic success. His brain gets the food it needs to perform, beginning with the most important meal of the day — breakfast.

Angie also notes that her son falls into a healthy sleep naturally after a day that includes exercise.

But Angie knows her son cannot be completely limited from doing the inactive things he enjoys, so she allows him to watch

Learn what to look for on the menu. Watch for low-fat options with words like au jus (in its own juices), baked, broiled, fresh, grilled, poached, lean, roasted, or steamed.

His mom, an athletic runner, says that's okay.

"I told Tim that's no problem. You can be an athlete without being on a team," Angie says.

On the other hand, Angie did insist that Tim become more active. There is no sitting around in their house in Harrisburg, Pennsylvania, where Tim lives with his mom and stepdad.

So, while his mom jogs every morning, Tim rides his bike next to her. They even turn it into a race to see who can go the fastest. Angie started this ritual when Tim was only six. It's so much fun that everyone forgets that they're exercising.

Tim is also an athlete on his own. Life is his sport. He will walk in the woods with friends. He bikes everywhere around town. He even bundles up on snowy days and bikes to the local YMCA.

Tim gets mostly As in school. His mom thinks diet and exercise play a big part in his

cartoons, play video games, or use the Internet for only an hour after he comes home from school. Reducing his screen time is a step in the right direction, leaving more time for healthy activities.

In Angie and Tim's household, good health does not begin and end with exercise. After Angie and Tim's father divorced, she remarried, and her new husband, David, is a vegetarian. The new family mostly eats a vegetarian diet. That presents some challenges when Tim visits his dad, who enjoys eating out on weekends.

Angie only allows a healthy menu at home, but she says her ex has "many different eating habits than what I do in my house. He eats out a lot. That is a challenge."

Suddenly, Tim, the boy who eats fruits, veggies, and salads all week will find himself at a fast food restaurant. The rules from his mother's home go with him to his

Quick Tips

- Try vegetarian foods as substitutes. Your kids won't notice if you substitute vegetarian "chicken" nuggets for greasy real chicken ones.

- Use healthy sauces like salsa on vegetables.

- If you're divorced, explain your food plan to your ex. Remind your child to eat healthy during visits with the other parent. Encourage them to eat salads and fruits if they're out to eat.

- Remember that an occasional burger or slice of pizza is a fun treat.

- Try not to serve dinner after 7 p.m. It might keep your child awake, and kids need sleep for good health.

dad's house. Tim tries to order salads with chicken and dressing on the side. He won't order something like apple pie for dessert. Instead, he orders apple slices with walnuts or low fat yogurt. He avoids French fries when his dad takes him out for burgers.

Angie says moms need to let kids know it's not the end of the world if they eat a few unhealthy things. She firmly believes that what matters is that you eat healthy most of the time.

She does suggest some tips to teach a child how to eat healthy when he's on his own. Angie told Tim to order his burgers with mustard instead of mayo. He asks for veggies on sandwiches, too. Many places will add lettuce, tomato, cucumbers, and even bell peppers or mushrooms to a burger if you ask.

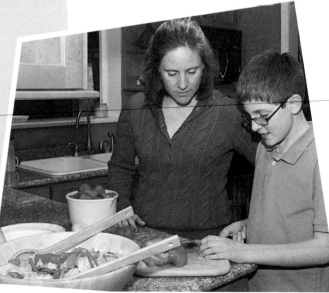

KEYS TO HEALTHIER LIVING

 Increase Fruits & Vegetables

 Increase Physical Activity

 Decrease Screen Time

 Decrease High Energy Density Foods

 Decrease Sugar-Sweetened Beverages

Tim's mom makes many vegetarian dishes for her family. They all love vegan chicken nuggets, which can be found at health food stores. They also eat black bean and veggie burgers.

Tim loves spicy foods so Angie will let him put salsa on almost anything, including eggs. Kids who love spicy foods often enjoy any vegetable with a little salsa on top of it.

For after-school treats, Angie buys low-fat soups. Tim also nibbles on natural microwave popcorn with no trans-fats. Mom says snacks don't need to be 400-500 calories. She makes sure Tim has 150-calorie snacks on hand.

Using logic and balance when it comes to diet and exercise, Angie feels that saying "no" all the time will only make a child want an unhealthy food more.

"Everyone deserves a treat," she says. "If the treat is fries once in a while, it's okay if you balance it out with healthy eating and exercise most of the week."

The family is about to expand soon. Tim's mom and stepdad are in the process of adopting a trio of children from India. They will add the siblings — two boys and a little girl — to this healthy, fun, loving household.

"I can't wait until they get here," Tim says. "They will have a family. I'll be a big brother. And I'll get even more exercise by playing with them!"

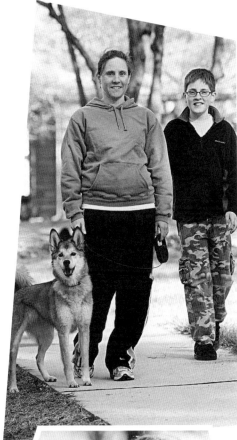

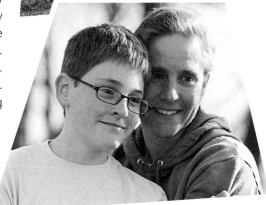

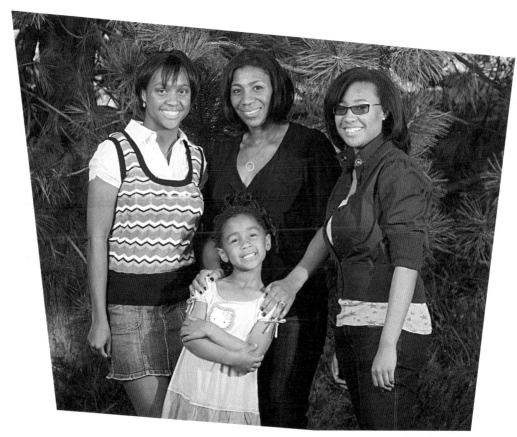

Gaye – Denver, CO

A MESSAGE FROM SUSAN

It took a mom in Denver to teach all of us that you can climb any mountain, so to speak, when it comes to incorporating healthy habits into your family's routine. Gaye is a busy parent to two teenagers, Taylor, 16; and Rachel, 18; plus little Mya, 8. Once overweight herself, Gaye made a commitment to not only change her own body, but to make sure that her daughters didn't suffer from the awkwardness and potential health problems of obesity and an inactive lifestyle.

Gaye doesn't just talk about good health, but puts it into practice with clever ways to make healthy, vitamin dense recipes that sneak in the nutrition. She also gets out there with the girls and uses the mountainous Red Rocks area of Colorado as their gym with mom working out just as hard as the girls. There is no better way to get your heart pumping than to do it together.

No matter where she is, this mom soars in all areas.

KEYS TO HEALTHIER LIVING

Increase
Fruits & Vegetables

Increase
Physical Activity

Decrease
Screen Time

Decrease
High Energy
Density Foods

Decrease
Sugar-Sweetened
Beverages

From the window of her Denver home, the snow-capped Rocky Mountains are visible, but Taylor doesn't notice. The 16-year-old is too busy making turkey tetrazzini with peas, whole grain noodles, garlic, and tuna. Her younger sister, Mya, 8, can't wait.

There is no candy or soda in this house. Little Mya gets graham crackers and whole-wheat snacks, which are much lower in fat than cookies, as treats. Rachel, 18, goes along with the routine, which includes cantaloupes and apples as snacks.

"We only eat junk as a treat," Taylor explains. "We read cookbooks, but cut the fat in half. We use much less oil. We even cut up raw potatoes in slices. Then you put them on a cookie sheet, spray them with a little olive oil, and bake them. That's a healthy French fry."

The woman who taught her daughters so well is a hands-on mom named Gaye, a petite powerhouse who once weighed 220 pounds. She takes veggies like broccoli and cauliflower and then whips them into a puree in the food processor. Then she puts that liquid into healthy whole-wheat mac and cheese or in spaghetti sauce. She even makes dark chocolate brownies (with the secret cauliflower puree in them).

Gaye's motto is simple: "Little food changes plus exercise make big changes," she says.

She also insists on everyone in the family eating breakfast. But, she adds, a fruity, sugary toaster snack is not breakfast. Neither is leftover pizza. Gaye refuses to start the day off on the wrong nutritional note. She makes muffins with protein powder and limited sugar in them. She flavors the muffins with different low-fat yogurts instead of using a lot of butter or oil.

Another small change she made is insisting that every meal and every snack include a protein and a carb. A great snack is apples with peanut butter. Almonds (protein plus fat) in yogurt (carb) also works, as does cheese (fat) with a few slices of turkey (protein) and a rice cracker (carb). Low fat granola (carb) with nuts (protein) in it also covers the requirement.

School lunches are a big concern for this mom. She suggests meeting with the people in charge of school cafeterias and asking them to serve healthy food choices, which has not only helped her children, but the entire school community.

Pizzas and bagels for school lunch aren't solutions for Gaye. She knows that children will get sleepy during their afternoon lessons if they eat that for lunch. It's not the child's fault. "You can't expect a child eating that much sugar to stay awake all afternoon," Gaye says.

Dinner is an adventure in Gaye's house. The kids don't even know what mom has packed into some of the dishes. She is a big believer in purees and will make a butternut squash puree and pour it into soups or stews. It's a great way to add in the veggies.

Gaye says that eating this way has helped her drop some unwanted pounds she once packed on a 220-pound body. These days

Cut back on beverages and foods with added sugars.

- Read cookbooks, but experiment. Cut the sugar and fat in them in half. The food will taste just as good. Soon your taste buds will require less sugar and salt, too.

- Keep soda in the garage so it's not handy.

- Along with regular daily exercise, set aside a special exercise day or night with your family. Ask the kids to find a great exercise and then show it to the entire family.

- Don't be the food police at home. Kids will resent it. Just keep lines of communication open. Let kids slip up. But on a daily basis make sure it's healthy foods that are served.

- Tell your children that it's great to teach their friends about their healthy habits.

she weighs 155 pounds. "Eating right as I came into my 40s was key," she says. "I was afraid of cancer. My family has a history of the disease. It was also about vanity. I knew I had to make these major changes."

Her children drink 100 percent juices and water, not soda. In fact, Gaye has never allowed her five year old to taste soda. But, being realistic, she lets her teens have chips and pizza at parties.

Gaye says exercise is key in her family and suggests walking with your children as a beginning exercise. She says that Mom's participation is very important. It's just the motivation kids need to get out the front door when they're feeling a little lazy. Her entire family will drive to Red Rocks, a free nature area by their home, and work out together. Mom is often the first one to lead a hike or climb the stairs. She can often be found running with her daughter, Taylor, and they pace each other to make sure there is a challenge to the workout.

"Believe me, it raises your heart rate!" she explains. "We drop to the ground and do push-ups. We'll do squats. We do lunges. You can do so much without a gym. Anyone can do what I'm doing in their own public park – and its free!"

At home, they have special exercise nights. Rachel loves to do yoga and dance. Taylor is into running like her mom.

"You just keep going," says Gaye. "That's the secret to life."

KEYS TO HEALTHIER LIVING

Increase
Fruits & Vegetables

Increase
Physical Activity

Decrease
Screen Time

Decrease
High Energy
Density Foods

Decrease
Sugar-Sweetened
Beverages

The American Heart Association recommends introducing healthy foods and continuing to offer them if they're initially refused.

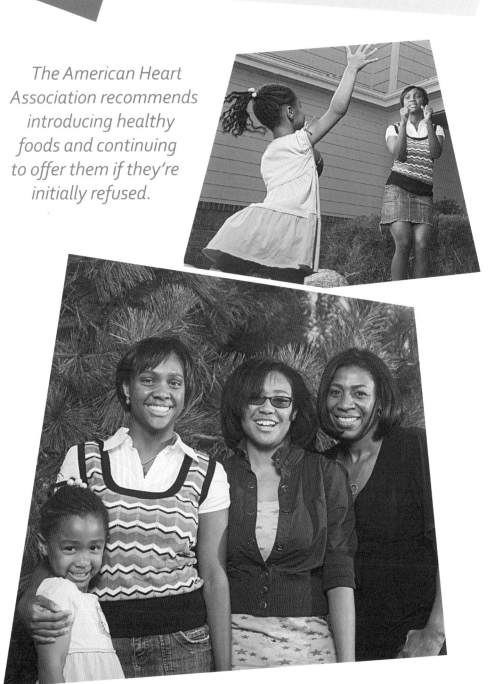

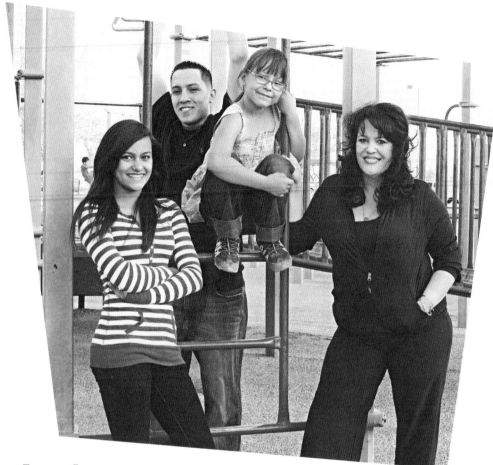

Andrea – Tucson, AZ

A MESSAGE FROM SUSAN

Andrea is a mother who touches my heart. She suffered a tragic loss when she lost her beloved baby son to cancer. Many women would crumble from this type of pain, but Andrea is amazing in the way that she healed and then made a special vow. This mother of three other children — Mickey, 20; Desiree, 12; and Alex, 6 — promised that she would do everything she could to make sure they lived the healthiest lives possible.

Andrea knows you can't prevent all diseases, but there are many health issues that are preventable with smart eating and exercise choices. The Tucson native faced a major challenge in her quest, which was her Mexican heritage. Andrea told me that her native foods are delicious, but so full of fat and salt that she needed to make some adjustments — ones that didn't always sit well with the older generation of her family.

I'm thrilled to share the story of this strong, smart, giving mother who never backs away from a challenge.

KEYS TO HEALTHIER LIVING

Increase
Fruits & Vegetables

Increase
Physical Activity

Decrease
Screen Time

Decrease
High Energy
Density Foods

Decrease
Sugar-Sweetened
Beverages

For Tucson mom Andrea, a life of hope was born of personal tragedy.

A woman whose family has lived for 43 years in the southern Arizona city close to the Mexican border, she comes from a culture that considers food an extension of love.

The family she raises in Tucson includes a now-grown son and two daughters. Roman, her first son, died of cancer as a toddler.

His mother's eyes fill with tears as she remembers her loss.

"Losing a son broke my heart," she says, tears streaming down her face. "Motherhood and raising my other children is the only way I survived. The kids who are still with me need

"Losing my son made me appreciate how life is fragile," she says. "Roman's passing away was a very sad life lesson. The lesson was to live life in the best way possible, which means you need your health."

Roman was diagnosed with a rare form of cancer. Trying to cure him took many surgeries and therapies that did not work. "He carried on for a year and a half," Andrea says. "He was so weak. But he would still smile at his mommy. Then one day without saying a word, he closed his eyes. He said goodbye."

Contributing to the heartache, Andrea's grandmother died a week to the day after she lost her son. Mounting medical expenses,

To get the nutrients you need, choose foods like vegetables, fruits, whole-grain products, and fat-free or low-fat dairy products most often.

my love. They need my heart and a good common sense approach to health."

Like many Mexican-Americans, in Andrea's family, food is a major part of their culture. The kitchen table is treated as a family gathering place.

While she always wants to honor her elders, Andrea also feels compelled to do what is necessary to achieve the simple goal of making sure her other children live healthy and happy lives. It's a vow she takes seriously every single day by changing their favorite ethnic recipes. Even when her older aunts raise an eyebrow at the changes, she reminds them that health is the most important thing in her world.

a divorce, and the need to get a job left the grieving mother with little choice. She moved into her late grandmother's house in a neighborhood that is considered one of the worst in Tucson.

The last thing on her mind was exercise and healthy food. It was hard enough just getting out of bed. Andrea worked two jobs and went to school. She faced a stack of bills at home. They lived on a diet of one pound of ground meat that had to feed both mom and son for an entire week. Eventually, she remarried, graduated, and had two daughters.

When life got better, Mom vowed not to take good health for granted. She got rid of

Quick Tips

- Take favorite ethnic recipes and make them healthier without sacrificing taste. Instead of frying beans in lard, you can steam them in a slow cooker.

- Use low-fat cheeses for recipes and cut the amount of cheese in half.

- If you know in your heart that a food isn't healthy, then avoid feeding it to your child on a regular basis.

- Change the conversation with your teenage children – talk about health instead of weight. Advise them about eating and exercising for good health.

- Limit or ban video games from the house for younger kids. Encourage kids to walk, run, ride a bike, or swim.

- Encourage your kids to sign up for sports — if they don't like it, they can always try something else. In most cases, the kids end up loving it.

any fast food knowing that she wouldn't give her children foods that were unhealthy.

There would be no more taco feasts like the ones she grew up with as a little girl. No more cooking in lard. No more high-fat cheese. It was hard because so many foods in her culture are cooked in lard.

Instead, Andrea bought a slow cooker for $30 and decided to find a way to make healthier Mexican meals. Now she puts whole beans in the slow cooker with a little water to cook slowly all day long until they're soft and ready to eat. Add some green chilies and spices like bay leaves and garlic to the mix and dinner is spiced just right.

Now, when Andrea, her husband, and the kids come home in the late afternoon, dinner is already cooking in three slow cookers. Soft, low-carb taco shells, spinach leaves, and lean meats are now on her menu. Tomatoes or homemade salsa, grated carrots, and radishes add to the flavor. She uses raw vegetables for dipping in guacamole.

The family garden includes tomatoes, onions, jalapeno peppers, peppermint, spearmint, chilies, and cilantro, which her children help plant.

When the kids get thirsty, Andrea serves them homemade iced tea instead of soda. A pitcher costs only 12 cents to make. For treats, there is air-popped popcorn made at home.

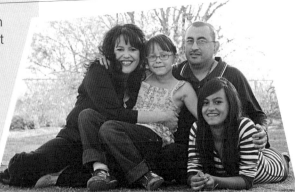

KEYS TO HEALTHIER LIVING

Increase
Fruits & Vegetables

Increase
Physical Activity

Decrease
Screen Time

Decrease
High Energy
Density Foods

Decrease
Sugar-Sweetened
Beverages

Cut back on foods containing partially hydrogenated vegetable oils to reduce trans fat in your diet.

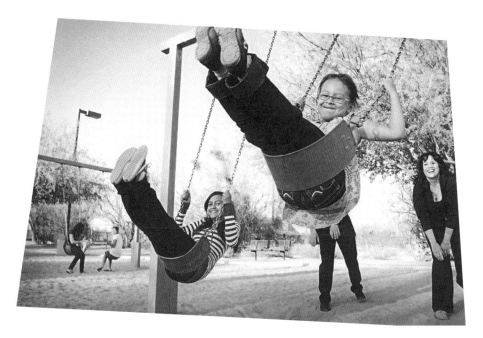

The tradition of cooking with her mother and great-aunts is now carried on with Andrea and her children. At her side, they have learned that burritos and enchiladas can be made in a healthy way by grilling chicken or meat after soaking them in lemons, vegetables, and juices. Even the older aunts agree that the changes are for the best.

Cooking with her kids has also allowed Andrea to carry on family traditions.

"Teaching them to cook means they will continue the traditions of our culture. But I'm also breaking an unhealthy cycle by teaching them how to cook to feel strong," she explains.

Sitting down at the table is also a form of bonding. She says cooking together as a family means the children will eat what they cook. It's also a great way to sit down in a quiet place and share the events of the day.

"My son getting cancer wasn't something I could prevent. But if there are diseases like heart disease, diabetes, and obesity that I can prevent, then I'm the mom. I will make sure we're doing everything possible for good health," she says.

"My hope for our family? It's that Roman is somewhere looking down at us, and he is proud," says his mother.

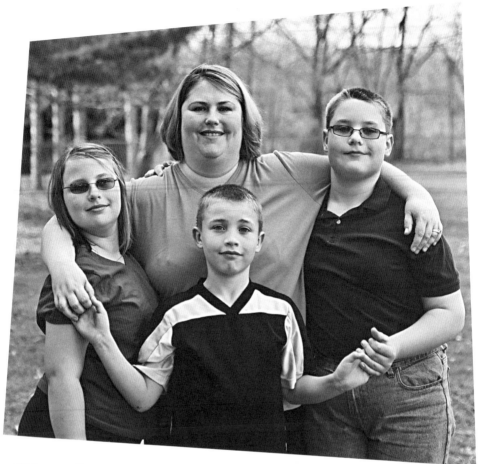

Cindy – Detroit, MI

I'm so proud of this family from Detroit, Michigan, because they define what it means to be a family.

When mother Cindy was diagnosed with type 2 diabetes, she called a family meeting that included husband and father, Dan, and their three kids Zack, 8; Samantha, 10; and Austin, 11. Cindy told them she realized that the lifestyle changes she needed to make in order to save her life were changes the whole family needed to adopt.

What were the biggest changes? They had to eat healthy, fresh foods and increase the amount of exercise in their daily lives. The kids didn't blink. They just wanted to know what they could do to help their mom. Now the family follows a healthy eating plan based on the Glycemic Index Diet. Mom allows the kids to have occasional treats, so they don't feel deprived. Cindy's goal is to make sure her family eats only the healthiest, tastiest food. She achieves it by mixing in a little fun.

KEYS TO HEALTHIER LIVING

Increase
Fruits & Vegetables

Increase
Physical Activity

Decrease
Screen Time

Decrease
High Energy
Density Foods

Decrease
Sugar-Sweetened
Beverages

There aren't many kids who are willing to give up a sugary birthday cake, but that's just what Cindy's son, Austin, did when he turned 11.

Instead, Austin, his family, and his friends feasted on a watermelon cut in half and decorated on the outside with pictures drawn with markers. The candles were stuck inside the juicy fruit.

"Our friends liked it, too. They came over and saw the watermelon cake and said, 'Cool!'" says his sister, Sam.

It was Cindy's diabetes diagnosis on February 16, 2007, that prompted major changes for this close-knit family. Mom, who works at the local emergency room, sat the kids down and told them that she was sick. She asked her entire family to help her get healthy again.

"I knew that without everyone's support, I would never make the changes. Austin was also a big kid. I didn't want him to turn out to be diabetic — and he was heading in that direction," Cindy explains.

Now the family practices the GI Diet (Glycemic Index Diet), and its basic principles are simple. Each meal consists of four ounces of low-fat protein, one starch, one fruit, and all the vegetables that you can eat. Grandma Patricia even created a special image on the computer of a plate with those requirements on it. The plate is always posted on the family refrigerator. It's a fun and easy way to remind the family of their meal-time goals.

After seven months, the entire family, including Grandma, had lost 200 pounds combined. Cindy alone lost 85.

"I can't even put into words how proud I am of my entire family," Cindy says.

The children were encouraged to try new foods like kiwis, Brussels sprouts, and spinach. When Austin wouldn't eat onions, his mother introduced him to sweet Vidalia onions. Now he loves them.

Cindy's kids even love liver and onions. Whipped, cooked cauliflower with a bit of butter is a substitute for mashed potatoes. Blueberries in plastic bags are a great snack for when the family's in the car.

Today about 1 in 3 children and teens (ages 2-19) in the United States are already overweight or obese.

When her kids complained about new foods such as asparagus or whole wheat grain products, Cindy asked them to try at least a few bites. Now, her children won't even touch a product that contains enriched white flour.

She also reminded the kids that peas, corn, and potatoes are starchy and should be eaten in moderation.

Cindy's kids have also adjusted to the sugar-free and healthier treats that are available in the house. No one complains about the sugar-free candies sometimes served for dessert. Besides fruit bowls, birthdays have also included cakes made out of sugar-free fruit gelatin topped with sugar-free whipped topping.

Quick Tips

- Ask your kids to try a new food three times before they decide if they like it or not.

- Make a game out of trying new foods three different ways for variety.

- Use the computer to keep programs on healthy foods and your eating plans.

- The only extras on the table should be vegetables. Dish out meats and starches at the stove. The family will eat less of those if the only second helpings available are the veggies.

- On Halloween, ask your kids if you can "buy back" their candy and give your child a penny for each piece. They can buy a toy they want with the money.

Another way they made eating healthy fun was creating a vegetable garden to grow cherry tomatoes, broccoli, onions, carrots, potatoes, and blueberries.

In this home, there is a "no fast food" rule. Instead, Dad cooks dinner at home with the kids if Cindy is at work. The kids take charge of stirring the sauce for spaghetti or making the salads.

When Austin, Sam, and Zack go to friends' houses, they're allowed to go off

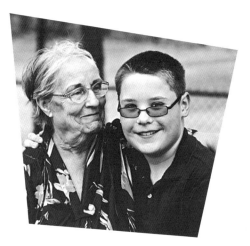

the diet, but not to go crazy. They prefer to only eat a little bit of a sugary treat now.

Once the family became familiar with this new lifestyle, they began to tell others about their success and how great they all felt. The children love to pass on the message about healthy foods to others at their school and in their community. Cindy has even started an e-mail newsletter, which she sends to friends and her own GI diet group in town. She shares great tips and recipes.

While the entire family has benefitted, Austin says the plan helped him lose 47 pounds in seven months. He

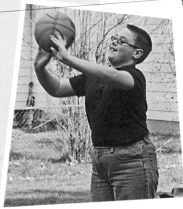

KEYS TO HEALTHIER LIVING

Increase
Fruits & Vegetables

Increase
Physical Activity

Decrease
Screen Time

Decrease
High Energy
Density Foods

Decrease
Sugar-Sweetened
Beverages

Overweight kids are more likely to become overweight adults.

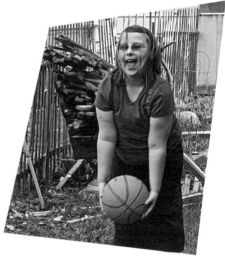

says the peer pressure for him to be thinner and look healthier was intense. His new lifestyle made shedding the pounds easy.

"I used to feel like I was the big guy, and that didn't feel good," Austin admits. "Now it's so much easier to move. I love to run, bike, and swim with my friends. I can actually beat everyone now!"

"This is a boy who used to walk slowly. He never ran. Now he runs, which is awesome," says his mother. "That was the

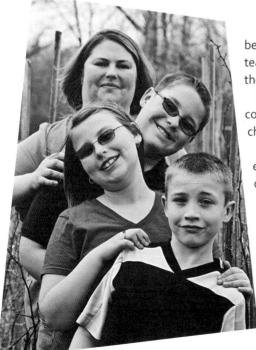

best feeling in the world as a parent. I had tears in my eyes watching him run through the yard the other day."

Now that Cindy's diabetes is under control, she has hopes and plans for her children.

"I want my kids to do anything they ever want to do," Cindy emphasizes. "I don't want there to be anything to stop them. They need to feel 100 percent all the time. The only way to do that is to eat healthy and be healthy."

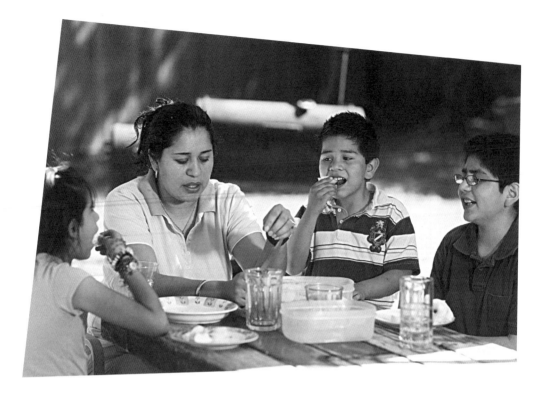

Emilia – Austin, TX

A MESSAGE FROM SUSAN

It's tough for a mother when she sees one of her children struggling. An Austin, Texas, mom named Emilia watched her oldest son, Sergio, 12, deal with a serious weight issue. She tried limiting his portions of food and suggested that he play outside. But her son loved TV and junk food — a very unhealthy combination.

Emilia, who is married and is also mother to Jessica, 8; Juan, 5; and Anthony, 3; didn't give up. She dug deep for a solution. It came in the form of a free community mission in her town called El Buen Samaritano. It's a place where families can exercise and learn new skills such as running, kickboxing, and even how to prepare low-fat meals.

The lesson Emilia learned in trying to help her son was that community resources are there for the taking. Why not get a little assistance from experts who are just waiting to help you? Joining El Buen Samaritano also led to a complete overhaul of this family's eating plan. They've gone from eating junk foods to healthy meals and now include exercise into their lifestyle.

KEYS TO HEALTHIER LIVING

Increase
Fruits & Vegetables

Increase
Physical Activity

Decrease
Screen Time

Decrease
High Energy
Density Foods

Decrease
Sugar-Sweetened
Beverages

Sergio was a young boy with a big problem — his weight. At age 11, he weighed 150 pounds.

Although he loved to compete in races with his classmates, he stood out among them. He was the largest boy in his class. Some of his classmates called him fat, and it hurt his feelings. Even when running in the races he enjoyed, he could not keep up with the others.

Tired of seeing her son disappointed when he came in last at every race, his mother, Emilia, set in motion a plan that would change the eating habits and recreational activities of her family of four children and of many others in her community.

Even Sergio's brothers and sisters needed help. But Sergio had the worst eating habits.

He hated vegetables and didn't try many fruits. The foods he loved included hamburgers, pizza, and big chunks of bread. Emilia tried to get him to eat smaller portions and to exercise, but he wouldn't listen.

Emilia's family, like many who struggle with money, spent a typical day eating, going to school, doing homework, watching TV, and eating some more.

"I knew this was bad for all of my children. For Sergio, it was even worse," she says. "I didn't know which way to turn."

She decided to reach out to her community by calling a local mission, El Buen Samaritano. Emilia heard that the mission offered classes in exercise, art, and healthy cooking. She had just never taken advantage of its free classes.

"Go out and look for programs that are free in your town," advises Emilia. "Go find your El Buen. These places are there. They're waiting to help you when it comes to your family's health."

Emilia suggests checking a local newspaper, listening to the radio, and searching online. Computers are available for use at libraries. Just type in "exercise for kids" and the name of your town during an online search.

African-American and Hispanic children are developing type 2 diabetes at much higher rates than their Caucasian peers. Almost half are at risk for developing diabetes.

Emilia says the next step is getting kids off the couch. At first, it was a struggle for her, so she insisted her kids come along when she went to El Buen Samaritano.

She also hid the remote control and told her kids that sitting in front of a television all day playing video games was bad for their health. When Sergio refused to take her advice, Emilia took him to El Buen Samaritano to do his homework. She did not give him a choice.

In time, it worked. Sergio joined the soccer and volleyball teams and liked them so much he began to enjoy physical exercise. Now he's the one who wakes up in

Quick Tips

- Get kids moving, either outside at a park or at a local club where regular exercise becomes a part of the daily routine for the whole family.

- Divide treats into small portions.

- Limit television and video game time, taking the remote control away and changing computer passwords if that's what it takes.

- As a mom, make sure you eat vegetables, too. Mention that you love how they taste because kids mimic their parents' behaviors.

- Make calorie guessing a game at home. Keep a calorie counting book on the kitchen table, so the kids can look up their favorite foods.

the morning and says, "Let's go!"

He even signed up for an activity at El Buen Samaritano called "Born to Run." And now he no longer comes in last.

As Sergio began participating in more activities, he watched his pants get too big and his energy levels soar. He lost 20 pounds while his mom, aware that diabetes runs in her family, began dance and exercise classes to get herself in shape.

But exercise was just one part of Emilia's plan. Healthy eating habits were also put in place when she began comparing calories in fast, fatty foods to those in healthy ones. She made guessing calories a game, convincing her kids to eat a 300-calorie healthy turkey sandwich instead of a 900-calorie greasy one.

She explained that a chocolate doughnut had 400 calories, but a cup of pretzels might only have 100. Calorie guessing contests and calorie charts posted on the fridge were

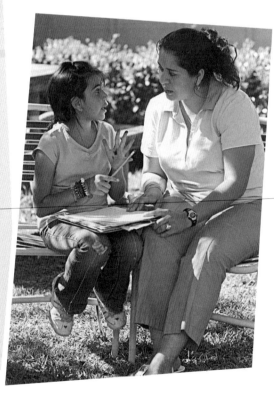

KEYS TO HEALTHIER LIVING

Increase
Fruits & Vegetables

Increase
Physical Activity

Decrease
Screen Time

Decrease
High Energy
Density Foods

Decrease
Sugar-Sweetened
Beverages

other approaches Emilia took.

Emilia got her children to understand that too much sugar is bad for them and asked them to compare food labels. She told them they would be better at their favorite activity if they cut the amount of sugar they ate.

It did not stop there. Emilia no longer allowed soda in her house. When she would permit it outside her home, Emilia would make the children split a single can of soda. The family went from eating hamburgers two or three times a week to having them once a week. Fruits and vegetables were added to daily meals, and her cooking was done with olive or canola oils.

Emilia feeds her kids dinner as soon as they come home from school because she believes they will eat more vegetables and healthy foods when they're truly hungry. She does allow snacks, but only healthy ones like grapes or low-fat popcorn without butter.

Emilia has noticed a lot of changes in her family and in herself. She has dropped two dress sizes. Sergio continues to slim down. He is excited to wear regular-sized clothes, and his behavior has even improved. The entire household rarely gets colds or the flu.

The children don't even want to watch TV much anymore. They would rather go to El Buen Samaritano to run and play.

"We've come a long way," says Emilia, proudly. "Our life has changed. We made good health a part of our routine. Eating healthy and moving is like breathing for us now."

"Our life has changed. We made good health a part of our routine. Eating healthy and moving is like breathing for us now."

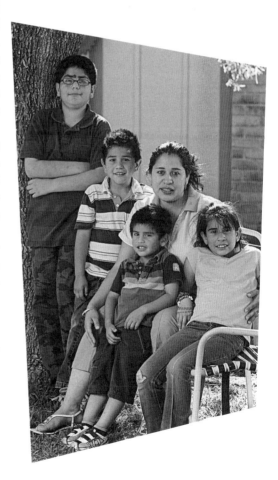

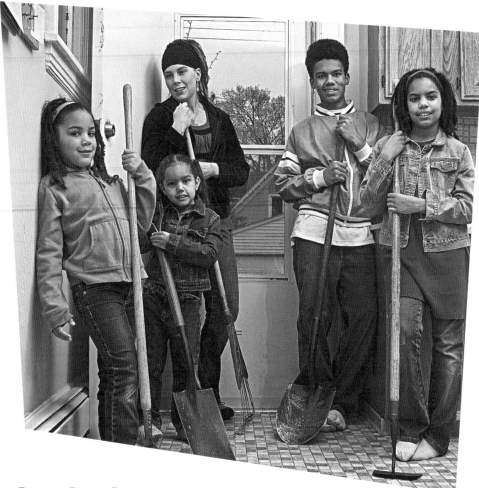

Christine – Minneapolis, MN

A MESSAGE FROM SUSAN

There's a Minnesota mother named Christine whose commitment to good health starts on the ground floor. She grows many of her fruits and vegetables in a community garden and in a space behind her new home in the heart of south Minneapolis. Her helpers? Her children.

Christine is a semi-vegetarian who worries about the pesticides found on grocery store produce. She knows that one way to ensure her children are eating fewer chemicals is to grow the food herself. It's such an inspiration to know that her children Jahdai, 13, Trinity, 10, Saba, 7, and Makeda, 5, each have pride in what they eat because they helped plant it, water it, and pick it.

Christine, who is also a busy nursing student, told us many wonderful ways to make sure what's on your child's plate is fresh and healthy.

KEYS TO HEALTHIER LIVING

Increase
Fruits & Vegetables

Increase
Physical Activity

Decrease
Screen Time

Decrease
High Energy
Density Foods

Decrease
Sugar-Sweetened
Beverages

Christine is a mother of four who doesn't just watch her children grow.

She watches tomatoes, kale, lettuce, zucchini, strawberries, and many other fresh foods grow in a miraculous garden outside of her new home in Minnesota.

It's not just that Mom has a green thumb.

Christine wants her children to eat from the earth. There is no better way to ensure this than growing the food in her backyard and in local community gardens.

"I know that our vegetables are the freshest possible," she says. "It's important to know what's on your food. I know there are no extra chemicals here. No pesticides. We plant seeds, water the young plants, and have our own harvests."

"It's wonderful to go outside, pick your food, and then cook it. You feel very energized and healthy," says Mom.

Christine is a semi-vegetarian who worried about the preservatives or toxins that cover many fruits and vegetables bought at the supermarket. So, she began growing her own food when she was pregnant with her oldest son. Seven years ago, she got involved with a local community garden.

She rents a small piece of land and grows whatever she wants in her space with her four helpers digging, planting, and picking ripe fruits and vegetables. In fact, sometimes her children can't wait and go ahead and rinse the strawberries with the hose and eat them right there in the garden.

Christine says it is an amazing feeling to participate in a community garden. Quite often, there is just too much food for one family to eat. "You share crops and become friends with your neighbors. I give lettuce and get squash. I trade kale for raspberries," she says. "It's also a good way to bond with your kids. We also get exercise working in our garden. It's so much bending and stretching."

She says that her children love working in the garden. Often they race Christine from the car to the plot of land. They wonder what has popped out of the earth and can't wait to harvest their plants. Naturally, they eat their vegetables because they grew them.

Only about 20 percent of high school students report eating fruits and green vegetables five or more times a day.

The other night her children were eating fresh raspberries that they grew and picked. It was much better than just opening a bag of cookies. Her motto at home is not to put junk in your body.

"I tell my kids that food is what we are," she says. "I ask them, 'Do you want to be junk?'"

Christine was raised on a farm and never enjoyed eating meat because she didn't like the process of killing the animals. This semi-vegetarian eats a lot of tofu, and she reminds moms that beans and rice together are great options to ensure your family's diet includes enough protein.

Limiting the amount of sugar in her house was a difficult task. While her children are

Quick Tips

- Start developing healthy eating habits at a young age. If you feed your very young children sugar, they will crave it. If you feed them fruits and vegetables, then they will develop a taste for them.

- Make food fun by growing a garden. Have your kids enjoy the process of a plant going from a seed to their dinner plate. Look for a community garden near you.

- Give kids a variety of vegetable options until they find what they really enjoy.

- Have a no-limit policy on fruits and vegetables. Kids can have "all you can eat" of these options.

- Find a local family restaurant. Call ahead and ask them to make a healthier dish for you.

allowed the occasional sweet treat, Christine tells her children that sugar is hard for their bodies to process and it blocks nutrients from being absorbed. She explains to them the benefits of eating fresh, healthy food and the impact the foods you eat can have on your body. "You have to speak to kids intelligently and give them facts."

Christine says the key is to limit the amount of sugar you give your children when they're very young, so they don't acquire a taste for it. When baking sweet treats, she often cuts down on the amount of sugar called for in the recipe or uses honey and other natural sweeteners as substitutes.

On the other hand, she says you should feed children a variety of fruits and vegetables from the moment they can eat solid foods. Children will become accustomed to them and will crave fruits and vegetables. Her own kids grab strawberries and carrots after school as treats. Mom doesn't even have to prompt them to crunch on celery or green beans.

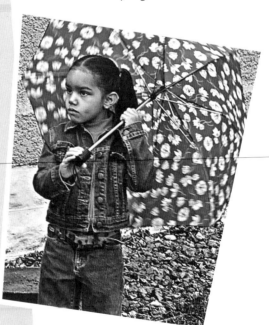

KEYS TO HEALTHIER LIVING

Increase
Fruits & Vegetables

Increase
Physical Activity

Decrease
Screen Time

Decrease
High Energy
Density Foods

Decrease
Sugar-Sweetened
Beverages

Serve a variety of whole fruits and vegetables daily, while limiting juice intake. Each meal should contain at least one fruit or vegetable.

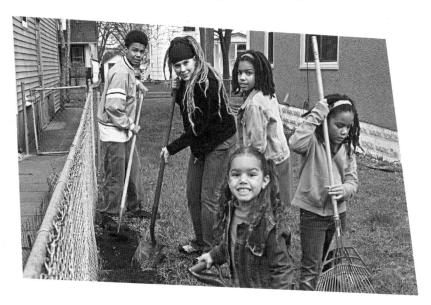

Her teenage son hangs out with his friends, but rarely eats fast food. He never developed a taste for it.

Most of all, she avoids prepackaged foods that contain many chemicals. Forget about finding those ready-made lunches in her kids' backpacks. She won't allow cereal bars because they have too many additives. She tells moms to look at the labels. If it has items you can't pronounce then put it down.

She saves money on the fruits and vegetables that she grows. Her community garden only charges $20 in fees and many of the seeds and small plants are donated.

The garden is a family-wide effort. In fact, Christine's son's first paying job was at community garden! Mom couldn't be prouder because she was the one who taught him how to plant his first seeds.

People often wonder how this single mom — herself a full-time student — finds the time to grow a large portion of her family's food. For her, it's simply a priority. She invests her time, because it saves money and it is an investment in her kids.

"My children are my inspiration. I feel secure that my children are eating healthy food and I'm passing along a great legacy by teaching them to grow their own foods," she says. "Kids love being part of the process."

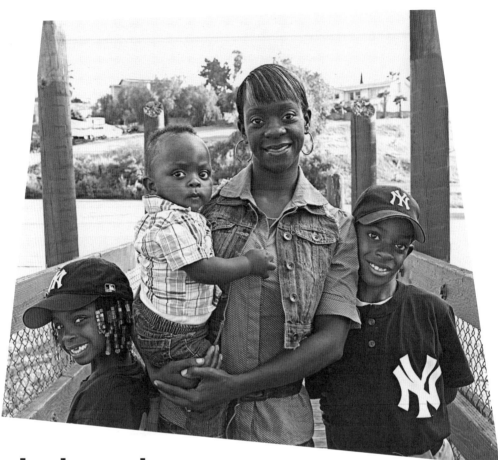

Lakeysha – San Diego, CA

A MESSAGE FROM SUSAN

Lakeysha is a no-nonsense mom in the best sense of the word. A former member of the U.S. military, she is just "Mom" to Elijah, 8; daughter Namaya, 5; and 9-month-old baby Victor. Lakeysha noticed that many children in her San Diego neighborhood were eating too much junk food and not exercising. To help the community and her own family, she began organizing events at a local park where the kids and parents can get moving in competitive and inspiring ways.

Lakeysha is teaching her children how to read labels and decide if what they're eating is good or bad for them. I love that she's helping them develop the food knowledge to make lifelong good nutrition choices. I like to think of Lakeysha as someone on the health front lines. The winners here are the children.

KEYS TO HEALTHIER LIVING

Increase
Fruits & Vegetables

Increase
Physical Activity

Decrease
Screen Time

Decrease
High Energy
Density Foods

Decrease
Sugar-Sweetened
Beverages

Lakeysha fought for the U.S. as a member of the Navy. Now the San Diego mother of three is taking on a different battle fighting for children's health.

A mom in motion who was originally from Chicago, Lakeysha served in the Navy's aviation administration for eight years in the California city that she now calls home.

"When I got out of the Navy, I knew my new passion would be childhood health and childhood obesity prevention. It taught me how important good health really is," says the mother whose young recruits know their orders come with love.

"It's important to fight for kids because they don't have a voice," she says. "Kids won't just say, 'I need to eat healthier.' Moms and dads need to step in."

Lakeysha says she hears too many excuses. But she has learned to ignore them and to fight back.

Every Tuesday, Lakeysha buys a local newspaper looking for food sales in an effort to save money and plan healthy meals. That's how her daily fight against greasy fast foods begins.

She taught her young children to read nutritional labels. Her 8- and 5-year-old kids even know about checking the sugar and fat contents.

At the grocery store, Lakeysha will take the kids through the aisles. The kids will grab a box of cereal and play this game. She calls it, "Is it healthy or not?" The kids will read the label and tell her, "Mom, we're not getting those sugar flakes. Too much sugar!" When they get to the produce, it's a big party. Her kids choose the fruit of the

Drink plenty of water each day.

week and pick the vegetables. Mom knows kids will eat what they choose.

Back in her kitchen, Lakeysha makes the cooking simple. Whole-wheat spaghetti topped with fresh tomatoes, rice and broccoli casseroles, and ground chicken and turkey are family favorites. When she wants to try something new out on the kids, she makes a game of it. To get them used to cauliflower, she let them taste it raw and then cooked. Everyone got to vote, and they selected the raw variety. The vegetable game has become a weekly event.

Her kids don't drink tons of juice because the sugar in the drink can harm their teeth. Instead, she uses plain or flavored waters. Actual fruits are turned into sweet treats, one for breakfast, two for lunch, and one when they come home from school.

Cookies are an extra special treat and belong in what she calls "now and then" foods. They are only served once in a while.

The end result is that her kids are spreading the news and helping other families with simple ways to get healthier. "When they see their friends eating an unhealthy lunch, my kids will say, 'That's not healthy,'" says this proud mom. "I guess they have me to blame."

Exercise is very important to Lakeysha, whose family has a history of diabetes. Her beloved grandfather, grandmother, and mother all have the disease. Mom knows that eating right is not enough to prevent

Quick Tips

- Search the Internet for healthy recipes. Go to your local library. Look at healthy cook books. Check them out. Seek out healthy ideas.

- Substitute water for sugary juices.

- At home, keep fruits and vegetables at a child's eye-level so they can reach for them as snacks.

- If you can't afford a gym, walk, use stairs, or run. It's all exercise.

- Teach by example by not bringing doughnuts or cookies to adult events. Instead bring a fruit or vegetable tray.

diabetes or other health problems. You must also exercise regularly to condition your body, burn fat, and act as an insurance policy against future illnesses.

"Kids are getting diabetes now more than ever before," she frets. It's just not fair that little children have health problems."

On the weekends, Lakeysha, her husband, and the children take hour-long family walks. She and her son run four times around a trail in the local park. Baseball, basketball, and football are other games the kids enjoy playing for exercise. The key is to make it fun, and the kids won't even realize that they just ran around for two hours or stretched their muscles.

"I never use the word exercise. It sounds like a chore. We go bowling. We go skating. Make it fun," Mom says. "It's better to go skating, wall climbing, or walking than to sit in a movie theater."

She says exercise makes bedtime easier, too. When kids get physical activity, their bodies crave rest and they nod off without much effort. This makes family life much easier for everyone.

Lakeysha spends her off-hours as a personal trainer and has set up a special exercise and nutrition program at her church called The Fit Club. She also runs her own nonprofit organization called Perfect Kids. To give back to the community, she organizes simple events at her local park, such as a basketball competition. She splits the kids into age groups and has them play for two or three hours with their friends. She will even give small, inexpensive prizes like a book or toy to the winners. It's a great way for the community to join together while the kids exercise.

This ex-military mom is no-nonsense about health. "I know about motivation and discipline from the military," she says. "Moms need to know that it's a fight to be healthy."

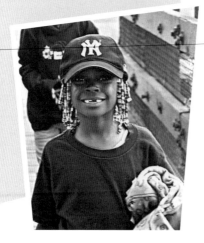

KEYS TO HEALTHIER LIVING

Increase
Fruits & Vegetables

Increase
Physical Activity

Decrease
Screen Time

Decrease
High Energy
Density Foods

Decrease
Sugar-Sweetened
Beverages

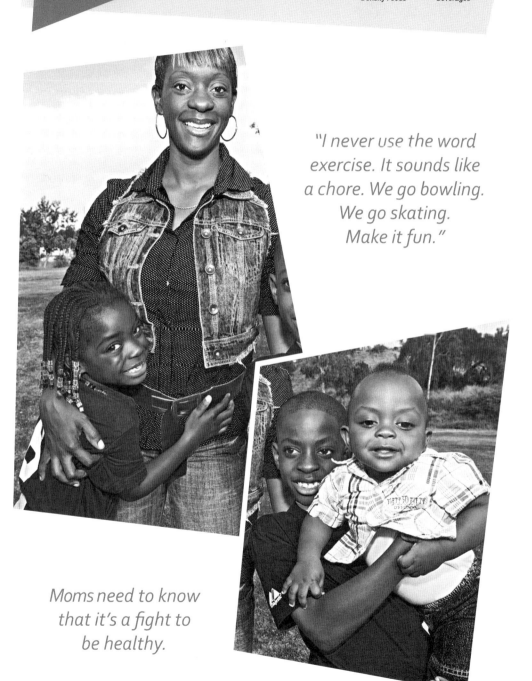

"I never use the word exercise. It sounds like a chore. We go bowling. We go skating. Make it fun."

Moms need to know that it's a fight to be healthy.

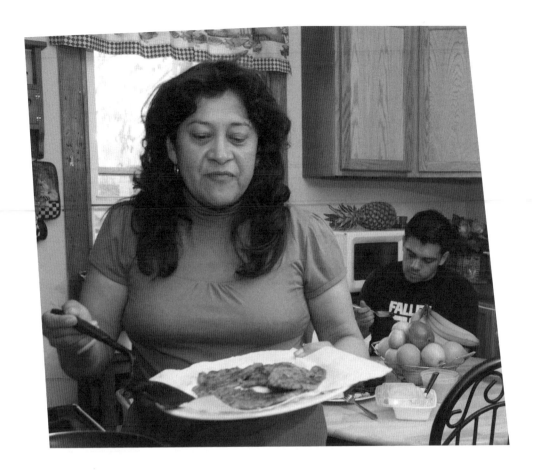

Jovita – Chicago, IL

It's never too late to learn life's lessons — or teach what you have learned. Jovita is a Chicago mother whose four children are ages 21, 19, 17, and 15. Her own father tried to learn about good health, but lost a battle to illness because of his bad diet choices. Jovita was diagnosed with the same health risks and decided to take immediate action. Knowing that she needed some help, she used free community health classes to learn everything possible about healing herself through food and exercise. She then made it a priority to change the unhealthy habits of her children.

Jovita's body responded in many positive ways, including weight loss and healthy checkups at the doctor's office. To give back to the community that saved her life, Jovita began teaching nutrition and healthy cooking through classes that are so inventive that word of mouth spread throughout the city. This mom gets an A-plus for her efforts.

KEYS TO HEALTHIER LIVING

Increase
Fruits & Vegetables

Increase
Physical Activity

Decrease
Screen Time

Decrease
High Energy
Density Foods

Decrease
Sugar-Sweetened
Beverages

A loving father never stops worrying about his daughter. Jovita found that to be true when she sat at her father's bedside in the hospital. He was dying of complications from diabetes, but grasped her hand and begged her, "Please, take better care of yourself."

Diabetes is a major health risk for this family. Jovita chose to ignore the disease until it caught up with her. Her doctors said she had a high risk and was already pre-diabetic. Watching her father pass away was like looking into a crystal ball and seeing an unhealthy future for her entire family.

Her father had problems with his kidneys, heart, and liver while also suffering from high cholesterol and high blood pressure. It was time to stop this unhealthy legacy.

"I was even more worried about my own children because our family has a history of these diseases," she says. "After my father died, I told my children that we all needed to make changes right now."

The changes she made were important ones. First, she cut out the whites — sugar and white flour. Her home became a "no fry" zone, and she used only a very small portion of canola oil to sauté foods and tossed out her lard. The meats she was told to purchase needed to be 95 percent fat free or she should use soy for recipes.

At first, her children weren't excited about following this new healthy plan. But Jovita was smart and involved them in only some of the new choices.

After teaching her children to read labels, she allowed her daughter to choose a breakfast cereal with natural ingredients including almonds, cranberries, and raisins.

Other changes were made without her children even knowing about them. Mom

Go with water, 100 percent fruit juice, or fat-free and low-fat (1 percent) milk instead sugary, high-fat drinks.

even scooted her kids out of the kitchen while she prepared some of the new foods to avoid any backlash. The kids didn't even notice the wheat pasta or soy that she added to recipes instead of beef.

"Kids will eat what you serve them. There shouldn't be any other choice but what the mother serves," she advises.

One day her son asked for a shake as a treat. She added oatmeal to low-fat yogurt and then tossed in fresh mangos. He never knew that Mom skipped the sugar or full-fat milk. He also missed the fact that Mom was now adding flax seed to the breakfast shakes and only a splash of real milk. The rest of what she calls her Crazy Shakes includes soy milk and fruit.

Her children always loved a high-sugar, high-fat Mexican dish that combines cornmeal, sugar, and chocolate. Mom decided to switch it around and mix brown rice, oatmeal, cinnamon, a bit of dark chocolate, and natural cane sugar. It turns

Quick Tips

- Don't just preach about good health in your home. As the mom, start eating healthier and model good behavior.

- Cut up fresh fruit and leave it on the kitchen table. Kids will eat the first thing they find when they come home from school.

- Find other moms and share healthy recipes and ways to cut out the fats and sugars.

- Start your own cooking classes in different homes with other mothers as a fun, inventive way to learn how to cook for your family's health.

- Healthy habits are formed over time. Start with small changes and gradually change your family's lifestyle.

Serve whole-grain, high-fiber breads and cereals rather than refined grain products. Look for "whole grain" as the first ingredient on the food label and make at least half of your grain servings whole grain.

out her children love the new dish even more than the old one.

A big victory was when mom was caught in the act. Jovita thought her son didn't notice that she wasn't making her trademark burgers without meat. This smart mom grilled soy patties so the burgers had lines on them and served them on wheat buns. She offered her children lettuce, tomato, and fresh avocado slices as toppings.

One day, all three of her sons brought home friends for dinner. Jovita told them there wasn't enough meat to go around for burgers. "I was so surprised when my son said, 'You have enough soy. We know you make soy burgers, and we love them,'" recalls Jovita. She didn't realize the boys knew her secret — or that they would enjoy the soy she added to the burgers.

Jovita's oldest son began to lose weight after living a childhood where he was always "the chunky one." One day, he came in after school and asked mom for a "green shake" made from peppers, zucchini, oranges, and soy milk because his weight loss had

KEYS TO HEALTHIER LIVING

Increase
Fruits & Vegetables

Increase
Physical Activity

Decrease
Screen Time

Decrease
High Energy
Density Foods

Decrease
Sugar-Sweetened
Beverages

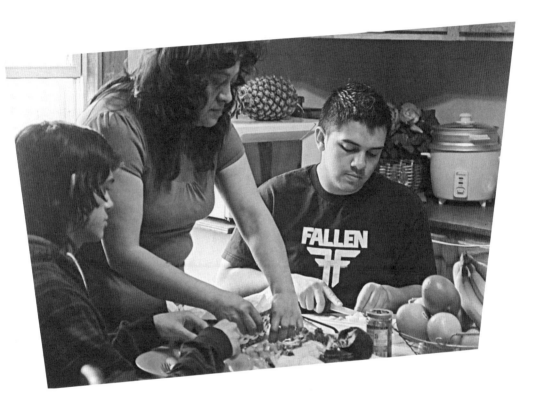

inspired him to be even healthier.

Once her family was on the right track, Jovita decided she would take her nutrition plans to the greater community. She gathered a small group of moms from her youngest child's school and talked to them about nutrition and good health. Soon, she was teaching several health classes around her Chicago neighborhood, including a cooking class. She's now made this work her career as a staff member at the Chicago Healthy Schools Project, where she teaches healthier eating.

Jovita's own diabetes scare is now under control through diet and exercise, and her children just received perfect checkups.

She knows her father would be proud.

"You have to pay attention to your health every single day," she advises. "My father made me realize that your health is the most important thing in life. I want to pass on the message that he gave me."

She knows it's not easy to change old patterns. "You just have to stick with it," she says. "Little by little your body will change a lot."

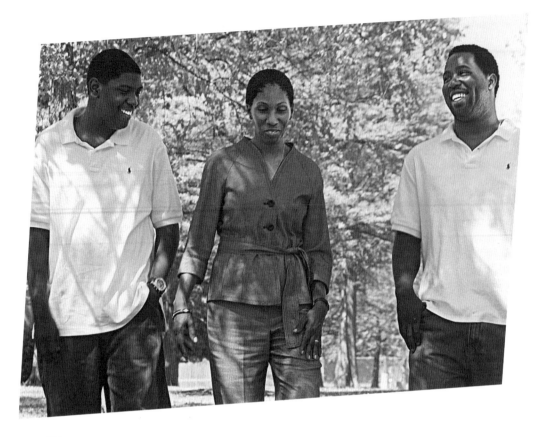

Sonora – Atlanta, GA

A MESSAGE FROM SUSAN

*S*onora is an amazing mother who lives in Atlanta with her two teenage sons and her husband Quavis Sr., who works as a police officer. Sonora was only 16 years old when she gave birth to their oldest son, Quavis Jr. Her younger son, Troy, was born two years later. Sonora faced every mother's worst nightmare when Quavis Jr. had open-heart surgery at age 15. Quavis Jr. survived, but doctors warned Sonora that she had to make some major changes for the health of her family.

Sonora is part of a loving family that fixes problems together. This household joined forces when Mom decided to change everyone's eating and exercise habits to help Quavis Jr. regain his health. This mom also wanted to prevent any future health problems by identifying their worst habits and finding reasonable solutions that would appeal to teenagers. Sonora made use of a great resource in her town that helped to keep her family members working out as they served as inspirations to each other and the community.

KEYS TO HEALTHIER LIVING

Increase
Fruits & Vegetables

Increase
Physical Activity

Decrease
Screen Time

Decrease
High Energy
Density Foods

Decrease
Sugar-Sweetened
Beverages

Sonora is a wise mother. She gave birth to her oldest son, Quavis Jr. when she was still a junior in high school. But don't let her age fool you. There is something inside of her that knows how to inspire children to be healthy.

When Quavis Jr. was only 15, doctors were forced to do emergency surgery to save the boy's life.

Following Quavis Jr.'s operation, his brave mother took command of the situation and immediately changed her entire family's lifestyle. She enforces creative solutions that don't cost much money and leads with pure determination. She's also the type of mother who takes control when times get tough.

"Sonora didn't just save our son's life," says Quavis Sr. "She saved all of our lives."

Sonora had learned that these types of health risks were related to poor diet and inactivity. She took her son's health problem and used it as a way to make her entire family feel better. She knew her biggest challenge would be changing the entire family's habits in order to help both of her sons grow up strong, healthy, and happy.

Quavis Jr.'s weren't the only health challenges in her family. Sonora's youngest son, Troy, was born with asthma. He was frequently rushed to the hospital when he couldn't catch his breath. Her little boy had to use an inhaler and was on steroids. He wasn't able to participate in any sports. When Quavis Jr. had his heart surgery, to Sonora it was just one more sign that it was time to stop these health issues once and for all.

Sonora decided the only way to make real changes was to lead by example. She wanted her sons to exercise, but the family had to be able to utilize resources that fit their budget. They would need gym memberships for four people. After years of volunteering at the YMCA, Sonora became an employee of a local Atlanta YMCA. She is proof that a place like the YMCA — where family memberships are sold at a very low cost — can benefit family

Being overweight or out of shape makes the heart work harder. Overweight children are more likely to grow up to be overweight adults and more likely to develop heart problems.

members of any age. Sonora can often be found on the treadmill working out next to her sons and husband.

Her sons had so much fun playing basketball and trying new climbing machines and weights that they didn't even realize they were working out. Sonora knew the key was going to the YMCA together as a family. No one wanted to be left at home when everyone was going to have a fun time.

Sonora also needed her sons to eat healthier foods. She is the first one to admit that she didn't know much about health when she married at age 18. Their diet as a young family was mostly hot dogs, burgers, doughnuts, candy, and deep-fried foods.

- Start your transition with a trash bag. Throw away the junk food in your house.

- Wait it out when kids refuse to eat. Kids will not starve themselves and will eventually eat what's in the house.

- Drink 100 percent juice or water to avoid salt and sugar.

- Replace red meat with skinless chicken breast, fish, and other lean meats.

- Use free resources such as a nutritionist at the local hospital to form a new eating plan for your family.

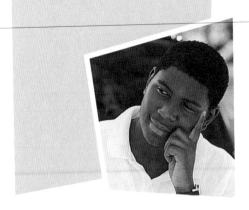

Sonora's father died of a heart attack at a young age and only ate these sorts of foods.

Eventually, Sonora became the family's guide on a journey to good health. She studied good nutrition and refused to buy foods that were processed or full of fat, salt or chemicals. While the man in her house missed the sweets and junk food, her kids had no choice. They ate what she served.

"You're the mother. You control the money and the shopping list. If you don't buy it, your kids won't eat it," she says. "That's the first lesson I'd like to tell other moms."

The next step was learning to cook in the healthiest way possible. Since cooking classes weren't an option, she searched the Internet and her local public library for healthy recipes. She found meals that were low in fat and high in flavor. Sonora also made good use of the nutritionist at her local hospital, a community service that is often free.

Sonora learned that she couldn't fry foods anymore. Her family learned to love baked and grilled chicken. Her secret is using garlic, lemon, pepper, and oregano on meats while avoiding salt. Sonora learned to buy only skinless chicken breasts instead of wings and thighs, since the breasts have the least amount of fat.

She also found a few tricky ways to make sure her sons ate healthier foods. Her sons said they hated skim milk. While she didn't like deceiving her sons, Sonora knew a little sleight of hand was required. She saved an empty full-fat gallon of milk container. When the boys weren't home, she purchased a gallon of skim milk and poured it into the full-fat gallon jug. Her sons didn't know the difference. A few weeks later, she told them that they had been drinking skim milk for weeks.

Her sons demanded white bread, but Sonora insisted they eat wheat bread

KEYS TO HEALTHIER LIVING

Increase
Fruits & Vegetables

Increase
Physical Activity

Decrease
Screen Time

Decrease
High Energy
Density Foods

Decrease
Sugar-Sweetened
Beverages

Check out the YMCA, health club, or recreational center in your neighborhood for a list of yoga classes, team sports, swim lessons, or other activities.

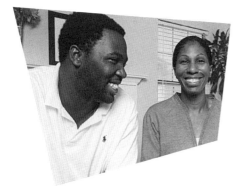

because it's healthier. It took only two days for the boys to give in to their mom. When they got hungry enough, they were in the kitchen making sandwiches on wheat.

Sonora and her husband continue to incorporate healthy habits at home. For instance, TVs were removed from the boys' bedrooms. They are only allowed one hour of TV a day in the den. This rule forces her sons to find other activities. Most of the time, the boys choose to spend more time at the YMCA, which earned them the title "The First Family of the East Lake YMCA." They're an inspiration for other families trying to figure out how to get more exercise. Quavis Jr. and Troy tell other kids about joining the YMCA and even invite friends to take advantage of trial memberships to work out with them.

Sonora's own health has improved because of her efforts. She talks about exercise and nutrition with other moms. She tells them how her own high blood pressure problem is gone now, thanks to exercise.

Sonora made amazing health changes for her family. Everyone is bursting with energy. Sonora and her husband lost weight and kept it off. Troy's asthma symptoms seemed to disappear. He doesn't even use his inhaler these days. Quavis Jr. has a strong heart and has just turned 18. He was even allowed to join his high school track and football teams.

"I love my children more than anything in the world," Sonora says. "I will do anything, read anything, buy anything, or try anything to help them be healthy. I want them to be successful and happy human beings."

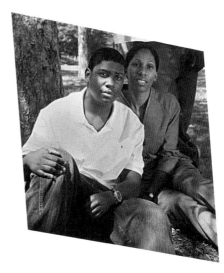

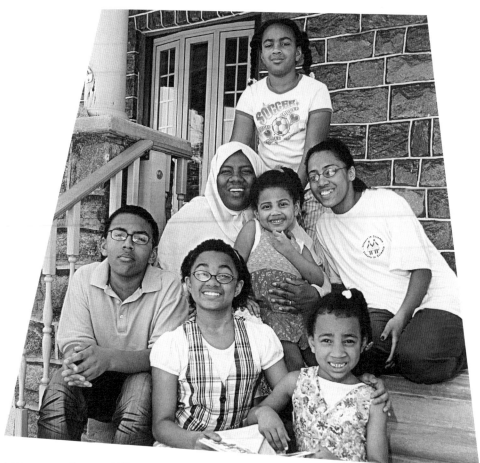

Rochelle – Philadelphia, PA

A MESSAGE FROM SUSAN

Rochelle is an inspiration who lives in Philadelphia. When it comes to her seven home-schooled children, she believes that good nutrition comes naturally. And she means that literally. She makes all of their meals the old-fashioned way — from scratch — because both Rochelle and her husband eat organic foods, as do their children: Armoni, 16; Cavhanah, 14; Adoniyah, 12; Keziah, 10; Keturah, 7; Bashira, 5; and Iman, 3.

Rochelle reminds us that, when our children are babies, we breast-feed them or feed them the natural formulas. So why feed them junk food when they get older?

When the temptation of bad, sugar-filled foods comes along, Rochelle is not afraid to say "no" to her kids. But she does it by offering a healthy substitute. Sound hard? Not the way Rochelle does it.

KEYS TO HEALTHIER LIVING

Increase
Fruits & Vegetables

Increase
Physical Activity

Decrease
Screen Time

Decrease
High Energy
Density Foods

Decrease
Sugar-Sweetened
Beverages

Rochelle is a mother who believes in doing things the natural way. She believes eating too many processed foods can lead to obesity and behavioral problems in children. The solution for her is as simple as the old rule of "an apple a day."

"If a child eats an apple, he will be healthy," she says. "If he eats those cookies filled with sugar and preservatives, he will be bouncing off the walls."

Rochelle is so committed to making sure her children eat healthy that it's almost a full-time job for her. She does the research and the legwork. Even on cold winter mornings, Rochelle and her kids walk to the local food co-op where natural foods are sold. She has taught her kids to get involved with community organizations that promote healthy eating. For instance, the kids recently helped educate their friends and neighbors about hormone-free milk by creating posters and promoting them at the co-op.

Rochelle wants her children to eat pure foods from the earth. She says that's the way human beings are meant to eat. "This is the most important lesson I'm teaching my children," she says.

There are no processed foods in her house, and Rochelle encourages other moms to use all-natural and, when possible, organic foods. One example of how to rid the house of the chemicals and preservatives found in cake and brownie mixes is to use multigrain flour and water to make pancakes instead of a mix.

Don't be fooled, though. Rochelle's family still enjoys sweet treats every now and again. To ensure her kids eat right, Rochelle has turned brownie making into an event, with one child measuring multigrain flour and another melting dark chocolate. That way she eliminates unhealthy white flour and sugar-filled light milk chocolate from the brownies. She also only uses about half the sugar called for in

Local parks are full of hiking, biking, and jogging trails that are perfect for families.

recipes and says her children don't even notice. Then she will "spice it up" by adding two teaspoons of vanilla instead of one and throw in some fruit for natural sweetness.

The "queen of extracts," as she calls herself, has a kitchen stocked with orange, vanilla, cinnamon, and even pineapple extracts. She adds orange zest from the peel of an orange to her baking.

Going natural is not as complicated as it sounds, according to the Philadelphia homemaker. Rochelle became a regular customer at a local farmers market. She thinks that's the best way to ensure that your children are eating healthy, with foods going fresh from the farm to the table.

To make sure her kids understand what she's teaching them, Rochelle takes them to local farms where the children can see for themselves how cows graze. Her children learn how vegetables grow and when it's time to harvest them.

- Moms should educate themselves on food content.

- Always find the freshest foods available. Visit a local farm so your children can understand how healthy food is grown and raised.

- When it comes to cooking, mix it up and spice it up, changing from lean meat one day to vegetarian meals the next. And be creative with spices and fresh fruits.

- When kids want to eat junk, have an alternative on hand. When kids ask for candy, give them maple syrup on oatmeal. When they want ice cream, give them strawberry yogurt.

- Encourage kids to exercise regularly by taking them to the local community center (like the YMCA), and by walking every place you can. Send your kids on an errand or have them walk to the store if it's safe.

In the kitchen, Rochelle works her cooking magic with low-salt seasonings for meats and unique spices or plain curry on chicken or fish. She also thinks the best way to make sure everyone's eating right is to buy whatever is in season, like apples in the fall and peaches in the summer. Eating fruits and vegetables that are out of season usually means they have come from far away and may not be as nutrient-rich.

For families who want to eat less meat and more vegetables, Rochelle suggests serving lean meat meals one day and vegetarian meals the next. For example, she will serve vegetarian beans with a salad

Let kids wash fruits and vegetables before cooking or eating.

for dinner. Or she will combine whole-wheat pasta with organic low-fat cheese and a splash of low-fat or fat-free milk to make a healthier version of mac and cheese. She even throws in a can of organic tuna to make sure her kids get protein in their diet.

Rochelle's simple approach includes homemade crushed tomato sauce over whole-wheat pasta, steamed vegetables, and fresh fish. When something healthy is expensive — like salmon for fresh salmon patties — she stretches it into two meals to serve her family of nine.

The end result of this type of eating is that Rochelle's own high blood pressure is now normal. She says no one in her house gets sick. Her kids are bursting with energy, but not bouncing off the walls. That's why Rochelle keeps it natural.

"We're creatures of this earth," she explains. "We need to eat in an organic, healthy way. It will keep you going strong for a lifetime."

Increase
Fruits & Vegetables

Increase
Physical Activity

Decrease
Screen Time

Decrease
High Energy
Density Foods

Decrease
Sugar-Sweetened
Beverages

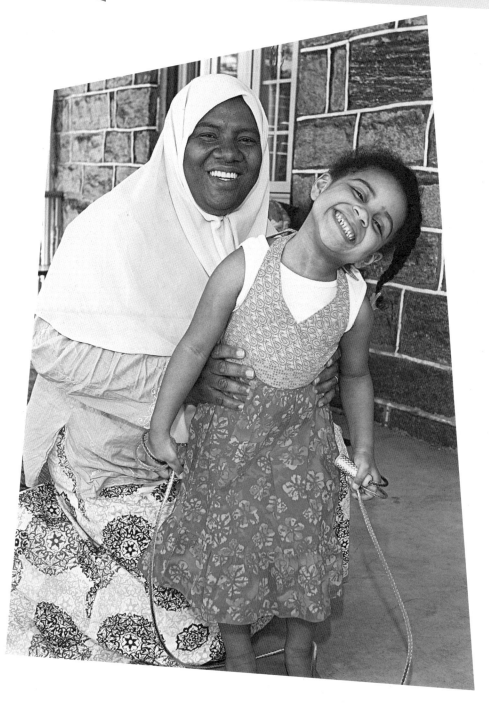

GLOSSARY

Additives: A food additive is any substance, other than the basic raw ingredients, used in the making of a food item to improve the final product. Additives are usually meant to preserve flavor during the production, processing, treatment, packaging, transportation, or storage of food.

Aerobic Activity: Aerobic activity (such as walking, bicycling, or swimming) temporarily increases your heart rate and respiration so more oxygen reaches your muscles. Aerobic means "with oxygen" and refers to the use of oxygen in the body's metabolic or energy-generating process.

Antioxidants: Antioxidants are chemical substances that protect against cell damage from free radicals. Free radicals are atoms or groups of atoms that can damage important parts of human cells, like DNA and the cell membrane. Well known antioxidants include vitamin A, vitamin C, vitamin E, carotenoids, and flavonoids. Antioxidants are present in dark green, leafy vegetables such as spinach and kale and may also be acquired through foods containing vitamins C, E, and carotenoids. Together as antioxidants, these substances are thought to be effective in helping to prevent cancer, heart disease, and stroke.

Artificial Flavoring: Artificial flavors are chemical mixtures that imitate a natural flavor in some way. Artificial flavoring is commonly added to processed food to improve flavor that has been lost in the refining process.

Artificial Sweeteners: Artificial sweeteners, also called sugar substitutes, are used instead of sucrose (table sugar) to sweeten foods and beverages. In the United States, five artificially derived sugar substitutes have been approved for use. They are: saccharin, aspartame, sucralose, neotame, and acesulfame potassium. Many people wonder about the safety of sugar substitutes but, with few exceptions, they appear to cause little or no health risk when used in moderation.

Balanced Diet: The American Heart Association (AHA) recommends that Americans eat a variety of foods including vegetables, fruits, whole-grain/high-fiber foods, fat-free and low-fat dairy, and fish twice a week. The AHA also recommends that people maintain diets low in saturated and trans fats and cholesterol and limit sugars, salt, and sodium.

Blood Pressure: Blood is carried from the heart to all parts of the body in vessels called arteries. Blood pressure is the force of the blood pushing against the walls of the arteries. Each time the heart beats (about 60-70 times a minute at rest), it pumps blood out into the arteries. High blood pressure, which is a health concern for many Americans, makes the heart work harder and increases the chance of a stroke, heart attack, and kidney problems. Diet-related lifestyle changes that can lower blood pressure are weight loss, reduced salt intake, healthy diet, and increased potassium (from diet), a diet rich in fruits and vegetables (8-10 servings/day), rich in low-fat dairy products (2-3 servings/day), and reduced in saturated fat and cholesterol.

Body Mass Index (BMI): Body Mass Index is a comparison of weight and height and is often used as a general indicator of health. BMI for adults can be calculated by dividing a person's weight by the square of their height (using metric measurements). The resulting score gives an indication of an individual's body/mass ratio. Scores can be interpreted as follows:

BMI	Weight Designation
<18.5	Underweight
18.5–24.9	Normal weight
25–29.9	Overweight
30 or greater	Obesity

Calcium: Calcium, an essential part of a healthy diet, is a silver-white metallic element that is an alkaline earth metal, occurs only in combination, and is an essential part of most plants and animals. Dairy products, such as milk and cheese, are well-known sources of calcium. Vegetable greens like spinach, kale, broccoli, and some legumes and soybean products are also good sources of calcium.

Calorie: A calorie is a unit of measurement for energy. For the purpose of measuring the amount of energy in food, nutritionists most commonly use kilocalories (equal to 1000 calories), and label the measurement either as "kcal" or as "Calories" with a capital "C". If that energy is not spent through exercise, unused calories can lead to weight gain. Approximately 3,500 unused calories results in one pound of weight gain.

Carbohydrate: Carbohydrates in food supply energy (calories) to the body. Sugars and starches (like potatoes, pastas, and bread) are types of carbohydrates. Whole grains are now considered the best source of carbohydrates (as compared to refined grains) because they contain the highest levels of nutrients and are high in fiber. They are also digested more slowly to keep your stomach fuller for longer and keep you energized longer.

Cardiovascular: "Cardiovascular" refers to the circulatory system (comprising the heart and blood vessels). The cardiovascular system carries nutrients and oxygen to the body's tissues and removes carbon dioxide and other wastes. Cardiovascular diseases affect the heart and blood vessels and include arteriosclerosis, coronary artery disease, heart valve disease, arrhythmia, heart failure, hypertension, orthostatic hypotension, shock, endocarditis, diseases of the aorta and its branches, and congenital heart disease.

Centers for Disease Control and Prevention (CDC): The Centers for Disease Control and Prevention (CDC) is part of the Department of Health and Human Services (HHS), which is the principal agency in the United States government for protecting the health and safety of all Americans. The CDC works to prevent and control infectious and chronic diseases, injuries, workplace hazards, disabilities, and environmental health threats.

Cholesterol: Cholesterol is a soft, fat-like, waxy substance found in the bloodstream and in all the body's cells. It's normal to have cholesterol. It's an important part of a healthy body because it's used for producing cell membranes and some hormones and serves other needed bodily functions. But too much cholesterol in the blood is a major risk for coronary heart disease, which leads to heart attack.

Chronic Disease: A chronic disease is a disease or condition that lasts for a long time. According to the U.S. National Center for Health Statistics, a chronic disease is one lasting 3 months or more. The leading chronic diseases in the U.S. include (in alphabetical order): arthritis, cardiovascular disease (leading to heart attacks and stroke), cancer, diabetes, epilepsy, and obesity. Health-damaging behaviors — particularly tobacco use, lack of physical activity, and poor eating habits — are major contributors to the leading chronic diseases.

Diabetes: There are two main types of diabetes, type 1 and type 2. Type 1 diabetes is something people can be born with, but type 2 (the most common type) develops in a person over the course of their life. In type 2 diabetes, the body has problems with a chemical called "insulin" that is important for the body to have the energy it needs to function. Overweight or obesity and physical inactivity are two factors that lead to a person developing type 2 diabetes. Over time if not treated, diabetes can cause problems for the body and increase the risk for heart disease.

Essential Fatty Acids: Essential or omega-3 Fatty Acids (EFAs) cannot be made by the body and must be obtained through the diet. The two EFAs are linoleic and ∝-linolenic acid. A lack of either will cause symptoms that can include scaly skin, dermatitis, and reduced growth. Such deficiency is very rare in healthy populations in the United States and Canada. Major food sources include certain vegetable oils and fish.

Fat: Fat is one of many essential nutrients. A chemical compound containing one or more fatty acids. Fat is one of the three main constituents of food (the others are protein and carbohydrate). It is also the principal form in which energy is stored in the body. Fat is the most energy dense macronutrient, containing 9 calories per gram. Certain types of fats are healthier for you (mono and poly unsaturated fats) while others are more dangerous to your health, "the bad fats" (trans and saturated). The American Heart Association recommends limiting consumption of saturated fat to less than 7percent and trans fat to less than 1 percent of total daily calories.

Fat Free: This means that there are fewer than 0.5 grams of total fat per serving.

Food and Drug Administration (FDA): The FDA is responsible for protecting the public health by assuring the safety, efficacy, and security of human and veterinary drugs, biological products, medical devices, America's food supply, cosmetics, and products that emit radiation. The FDA is also responsible for improving the public health by helping to speed progress that makes medicines and foods more effective, safer and more affordable; and helping the public get the accurate, science-based information they need to use medicines and foods to improve their health.

Glucose: Glucose is a simple sugar and the chief source of energy in the body. The body makes glucose from proteins, fats, and carbohydrates, then carries it to each cell through the bloodstream.

Heart Attack: A heart attack is a problem that can happen as a result cardiovascular disease when something blocks blood flow to part of the heart and the heart muscle begins to die because it isn't getting any oxygen.

Heart Disease: Heart disease, also called cardiovascular disease, means that there is a problem with a person's heart and blood vessels. Heart disease is caused by atherosclerosis (ath"er-o-skleh-RO'sis), the narrowing of the coronary arteries due to fatty build ups of plaque. It's likely to produce angina pectoris (chest pain), heart attack, or both. Heart disease is caused by several factors, know as risk factors. Some risk factors we can't do anything about (like your genetics), but other risk factors we can control, like not smoking, making healthy food choices, maintaining a healthy weight, staying physically active each day, and maintaining a normal blood pressure. Heart disease is the leading cause of death in the United States.

High Blood Pressure: Blood pressure is the pressure the blood in the body puts on the walls of the blood vessels (the tubes in the body that carry blood around) when your heart beats. Blood pressure increases when the heart beats and falls when the heart relaxes between beats. Blood pressure is impacted by activity, rest, temperature, emotions, diet and many other factors. High blood pressure is the number-one cause of a stroke.

High Cholesterol: Too much cholesterol in the blood is called hypercholesterolemia. This can create sticky deposits (called plaque) along the artery walls and may lead to heart disease and atherosclerosis.

High Energy Dense Foods: Energy density is the amount of energy (calories) per gram of food. Energy density measures the energy released when the food is metabolized after it is ingested and the food is metabolized with oxygen, into waste products such as carbon dioxide and water. High energy dense foods have more than three calories per gram and include crackers, cheese, dark chocolate, and peanuts.

High Fiber Foods: Foods that have 5 grams or more of fiber per serving are considered to be high-fiber foods.

Hydrogenated Fat: A fat that has been chemically altered by the addition of hydrogen atoms (see trans fatty acid). Vegetable shortening and margarine are hydrogenated fats. Like saturated or animal fats, hydrogenated fats contribute to clogged arteries. The federal government, dietitians, and other health professionals recommend limiting the amount of hydrogenated fats in the diet.

Hypertension: People whose blood pressure is above a normal range are said to have high blood pressure, or hypertension. Hypertension can increase a person's risk for cardiovascular disease because the heart and blood vessels are working harder than normal. Hypertension often runs in families – but maintaining a healthy weight by making healthy food choices and staying physically active for at least 60-minutes per day for children and 60 minutes for adults (over age 18) can help prevent hypertension, even with a family history.

Insulin: Insulin is a hormone that lowers the level of glucose (a type of sugar) in the blood. It's made by the beta cells of the pancreas and released into the blood when the glucose level goes up, such as after eating. Insulin helps glucose enter the body's cells, where it can be used for energy or stored for future use. If someone has diabetes, the person's pancreas doesn't make enough insulin or the body can't respond normally to the insulin that is made. This causes the glucose level in the blood to rise.

Low caloric density: The caloric density of a food is the number of calories that are contained in 1 gram of that food. Foods that contain .5 calories or less per gram are considered to have low caloric density.

Low-Fat: Foods that are low-fat contain limited amounts of fat. Typically, foods that contain 3 grams of fat per serving or less are considered low-fat.

Low-Sodium (Low-Salt): Foods that contain less than 140 milligrams or less of sodium (salt) per serving are considered low-sodium. The American Heart Association recommends that individuals limit their daily sodium consumption to 2,300 mg per day.

Moderate Activity: Moderate-intensity physical activity refers to a level of effort in which a person should experience some increase in breathing or heart rate. Examples of moderate activities are brisk walking, swimming, cycling, and dancing.

Muscle Strengthening Activity: Muscle strengthening activities build muscle endurance along with muscle strength. These activities help to decrease body fat and increase lean muscle mass. Increasing lean muscle mass can help your body burn calories more efficiently.

Natural Flavoring: These are natural flavors such as the essential oil, essence, extractive, or distillate that contains flavoring from a food (including a spice, fruit, vegetable, yeast, herb, bark, bud, root, leaf, meat, seafood, poultry, egg, or dairy product) whose main purpose is flavoring, not nutritional enhancement.

Non-Competitive Sports: Non-competitive sports are activities that occur in a recreational setting (like a playground, school gym, or schoolyard). These activities may have an outcome (win or loss), but don't lead to championships or tournaments and don't involve formal teams or documented outcomes (such as standings).

Nutrient-Dense Foods: Nutrient-dense foods are those that provide large amounts of vitamins and minerals and fewer calories.

Nutrition: Nutrition is the processes by which a living thing consumes food and uses it for growth and maintenance. Nutrition is also the scientific study of food and drink, especially in humans.

Obesity: Obesity is defined as too much body fat. Your body is made up of water, fat, protein, carbohydrate, and various vitamins and minerals. If you have too much fat — especially in your waist area — you're at higher risk for health problems, including high blood pressure, high blood cholesterol, diabetes, heart disease, and stroke. Obesity in adults is defined as a BMI of 30.0 or greater or about 30 pounds or more overweight; extreme obesity is defined as a BMI of 40 or greater. Obesity in children is defined as at or above the 95th percentile BMI-for-age.

Obesogenic: Something that leads to or promotes obesity can be referred to as obesogenic.

Organic Foods: According to the U.S. Department of Agriculture, organic food is produced by farmers who stress the use of renewable resources and the conservation of soil and water to improve the environment for future generations. Organic meat, poultry, eggs, and dairy products come from animals that are given no antibiotics or growth hormones. Organic food is produced without using most conventional pesticides; fertilizers made with synthetic ingredients or sewage sludge; bioengineering; or ionizing radiation. The USDA runs a National Organic Program (NOP) that provides standardized guidelines for organic foods.

Osteoporosis: Osteoporosis is a condition that results in thinning of the bones and reduction in bone mass. It is commonly due to lessening of calcium and bone protein. Osteoporosis makes a person more susceptible to fractures and is more common in older adults, particularly women. Osteoporosis can lead to changes in posture, physical abnormality, and decreased mobility. To avoid osteoporosis, doctors recommend a balanced diet including calcium-rich foods.

Overweight: Overweight in adults is defined as a body mass index of 25 to less than 30. A BMI of about 25 corresponds to about 10 percent over ideal body weight. Overweight in children is defined as at or above the 85th percentile BMI-for-age.

Pancreas: A long, flat gland located behind the stomach that secretes insulin and glucagon, which are hormones that control blood sugar levels, and digestive enzymes that are needed to break down foods so that nutrients can be absorbed by the small intestine.

Partially Hydrogenated Vegetable Oil:
Hydrogenation is widely applied to the processing of vegetable oils and fats. Complete hydrogenation converts unsaturated fatty acids to saturated ones. Typically the process is not usually completed, and the result is described as partially hydrogenated vegetable oil. Some, but usually not all, of the double bonds in each molecule have been reduced. This is done by limiting the amount of hydrogen allowed to react with the fat.

Pesticides: Pesticides are chemicals designed to protect crops. They are commonly subdivided into four types:
1. Insecticides are used to control insects.
2. Herbicides are used to control weeds.
3. Rodenticides are used to control rodents.
4. Fungicides are used to control mold, mildew, and fungi.
The federal government attempts to regulate pesticides to ensure that their use does not cause unreasonable risks to humans or the environment.

Physical Activity: Physical activity is any bodily movement produced by skeletal muscles that results in energy being used. The American Heart Association recommends adults get regular moderate to vigorous physical activity for at least 60 minutes a day on most if not all days of the week. Children should be moderately to vigorously physically active for at least 60 minutes everyday.

Portion Size: The amount of food presented in one eating occasion.

Preservatives: Preservatives are used to prevent food from spoiling. Preservatives sometimes increase the shelf life of a food and assist in keeping the flavor. Some processed foods that contain preservatives may have higher sodium (salt) or sugar than whole or raw foods.

Processed Foods: Processed foods have been specially treated or changed to create a new product, increase the shelf life of a food, or to make it easier to transport and store. Processing sometimes causes raw or whole-grain foods to lose vitamins and nutrients without reducing calories.

Protein: Protein is also a source of energy. Foods that contain proteins include animal products, grains, legumes, and vegetables. The USDA recommends that, when eating protein, most meat and poultry choices should be lean or low-fat. They also say that fish, nuts, and seeds contain healthy oils, so it is recommended to choose these foods often instead of meat or poultry.

Pulse: Your pulse tells you how fast or slow your heart is beating—also called your heart rate. The walls of your heart are made of really strong muscles that squeeze and relax to pump blood around your body. Your pulse is the number of times your heart beats each minute (what scientists call "beats per minute" or bpm).

Refined Grain: Refined grain is a type of starch that is less nutritious than a whole grain because it is more processed and has less fiber, vitamins, and minerals. Some examples of refined grains include white rice, white pasta, and breads that contain enriched-wheat flour.

Saccharin: Saccharin is an artificial sweetener. The basic substance, benzoic sulfinide, has no food energy (or fat) and is much sweeter than sucrose, but has an unpleasant bitter aftertaste, especially in large servings. It is used to sweeten products such as drinks, candies, medicines, and toothpaste.

Safe Drinking Water: Safe drinking water includes water from a bottle or tap that meets the Environmental Protection Agency's (EPA) standards for drinking. For more information about your city's water quality, visit the EPS's web site or contact your local water company.

Saturated Fat: Saturated fats are those that have no room on the molecule for additional hydrogen. Saturated fats are found primarily in animal products — red meat, lard, butter, poultry with skin and whole milk dairy products. Palm and coconut oils are also saturated, as is vegetable shortening and margarine ("hydrogenated"). Eating too many saturated fats is linked to higher levels of damaging cholestorol, heart and blood vessel disease, and many types of cancers.

Sedentary Lifestyle: A sedentary lifestyle means a person is inactive for most of the time. A sedentary lifestyle can lead to obesity, heart disease, or other health complications.

Serving Size: A standardized amount of a food, such as a cup or an ounce, used in providing dietary guidance or in making comparisons among similar foods.

Sodium (Salt): Sodium is a mineral and an essential nutrient for the human body. Diets high in sodium can lead to high blood pressure or other health complications. Aim to eat less than 2,300 mg of sodium per day. Some people — African-Americans, middle-aged and older adults, and people with high blood pressure — should aim for less than 1,500 mg per day.

Sugar Free: Foods that contain 0.5 grams or less of sugar per serving are considered to be sugar free.

Stroke: Stroke is a disease of the blood vessels of the brain otherwise known as cerebrovascular disease. A stroke occurs when a blood vessel that carries oxygen and nutrients to the brain gets blocked or bursts. When that happens, part of the brain cannot get the blood (and oxygen) it needs, so it starts to die. Without the right medical attention, a stroke can cause permanent damage to the brain and the body or even death. People most likely to have a stroke are over 55, don't eat a balanced diet, are physically inactive, may be obese, and have other risk factors for heart disease like high blood pressure, high cholesterol, or diabetes.

Trans Fats: Trans fat is a specific type of fat formed when liquid oils are chemically processed into solid fats like shortening and hard margarine. It is typically found in products that contain "partially hydrogenated vegetable oils," such as some salty snacks and commercially baked and deep-fried foods, although trans fat also occurs naturally in animal products such as meat and dairy products that contain fat. Trans fats and saturated fats (known as the "bad fats") are both associated with an increased risk of heart disease because

they raise the levels of total blood cholesterol and LDL cholesterol (low-density lipoproteins or "bad" cholesterol). Unlike saturated fats, trans fats may also lower HDL cholesterol (high-density lipoproteins or "good" cholesterol). The AHA recommends consuming less than 1 percent of your calories from trans fat each day or less than 2 g for someone who needs 2,000 calories each day.

Type 1 Diabetes: Type 1 diabetes (insulin dependent diabetes), also know as "juvenile diabetes," occurs when the pancreas can't make enough insulin for the body. Type 1 diabetes often begins in childhood or the young adult years, but people of any age can get it. It is less common than Type 2 and is often attributed to genetics.

Type 2 Diabetes: Non-insulin dependent (Type 2) diabetes is the most common type of diabetes and develops slowly over time. Traditionally, type 2 diabetes occurred after age 40, but today it is being found more often among younger Americans. Diabetes is often associated with obesity or high levels of cholesterol. Type 2 diabetes can often be prevented and controlled through diet, weight control, and exercise.

Unsaturated Fats: Unsaturated fats are fat molecules with double bonds, which have room for additional hydrogen. Monounsaturated fats can bond two additional hydrogen atoms and polyunsaturated fats can bond more hydrogen atoms. Unsaturated fats are usually found in plant products, like vegetable oils such as peanut, canola, and olive (monounsaturated) and sunflower, corn, and safflower (polyunsaturated). Fish oils are unique as animal sources of polyunsaturated fat. Unsaturated fats have been shown to reduce cholesterol levels in some individuals, which may reduce risk of heart disease.

Vigorous Activity: Vigorous-intensity physical activity may be intense enough to lead to a large challenge to an individual and refers to a level of effort in which a person should experience a large increase in breathing or heart rate and sweating. Examples of vigorous physical activities include jogging/running, lap swimming, cycling, aerobic dancing, skating, rowing, jumping rope, cross-country skiing, hiking/backpacking, racquet sports, and competitive group sports (for example, soccer and basketball).

Whole Grains: Foods made from an entire grain seed (usually called the kernel), which consists of the bran, germ, and endosperm. Whole-grain foods contain more nutrients than refined grain food.

For more messages from moms on living healthier lives, information childhood obesity, tips for healthy living, or to submit your own story, please visit the Be Well web site at **www.bewellbook.org.**

For more information on the organizations and resources discussed in this book, please visit the web sites listed below:

Alliance for a Healthier Generation
www.HealthierGeneration.org

American Heart Association
www.americanheart.org

Centers for Disease Control and Prevention
www.cdc.org

El Buen Samaritano (Austin, TX)
www.elbuen.org

Healthy Schools Campaign (Chicago, IL)
www.healthyschoolscampaign.org

Michael & Susan Dell Foundation
www.msdf.org

My Pyramid
www.MyPyramid.gov

William J. Clinton Foundation
www.clintonfoundation.org

YMCA of America
www.ymca.org

ACKNOWLEDGEMENTS

This book is entirely about people. There are so many important people that have made this book possible. I extend my sincere thanks to the individuals and organizations that have contributed to this project.

Thank you to our partner in this endeavor, the Alliance for a Healthier Generation, a partnership between the American Heart Association and the William J. Clinton Foundation.

This book began as an idea. The finished product is a result of the amazing work by dedicated individuals: Janet Mountain, Megan Matthews, Dr. Aliya Esmail Hussaini, and members of the phenomenal staff at the Michael & Susan Dell Foundation.

We appreciate all of the moms — or people who knew an inspirational mom — who told us their stories and inspired us to help others lead healthier lives. There are so many organizations in the United States committed to combating childhood obesity and to helping families, and they were our greatest assets as we scoured the United States in search of the stories to feature in this book. Those organizations that went above and beyond to assist us include: El Buen Samaritano in Austin, TX; the Food Trust in Philadelphia, PA; the Harlem YMCA in New York, NY; the Healthy Schools Campaign in Chicago, IL; the Midtown YWCA in Minneapolis, MN; the Network for a Healthy California; the Parent Academy in Miami, FL; the Shih Yu-Lang Central YMCA in San Francisco, CA; the South Chicago YMCA in Chicago, IL; the Villages at Carver YMCA in Atlanta, GA; and the YMCA Teen Center in Oakland, CA.

We are grateful to the people who took some words and brought the book to life: KariAnne Harmon, Amy Robinson, and Erica Espiritu at American Airlines Publishing provided much needed counsel and guidance, and Angela Austin Dake at Weber Shandwick whose dedication to finding our moms was second to none.

Most importantly, our deepest gratitude is extended to the amazing women whose stories are included in this book. Thank you for sharing your lives with us so others might lead healthier ones.

— Susan Dell
2009

Thank you for sharing your lives with us so that others might lead healthier ones.